Health Care Evaluation

Understanding Public Health

Series editors: Nick Black and Rosalind Raine, London School of Hygiene & Tropical Medicine

Throughout the world, recognition of the importance of public health to sustainable, safe and healthy societies is growing. The achievements of public health in nineteenth-century Europe were, for much of the twentieth century, overshadowed by advances in personal care, in particular in hospital care. Now, with the dawning of a new century, there is increasing understanding of the inevitable limits of individual health care and of the need to complement such services with effective public health strategies. Major improvements in people's health will come from controlling communicable diseases, eradicating environmental hazards, improving people's diets and enhancing the availability and quality of effective health care. To achieve this, every country needs a cadre of knowledgeable public health practitioners with social, political and organizational skills to lead and bring about changes at international, national and local levels.

This is one of a series of 20 books that provides a foundation for those wishing to join in and contribute to the twenty-first-century regeneration of public health, helping to put the concerns and perspectives of public health at the heart of policy-making and service provision. While each book stands alone, together they provide a comprehensive account of the three main aims of public health: protecting the public from environmental hazards, improving the health of the public and ensuring high quality health services are available to all. Some of the books focus on methods, others on key topics. They have been written by staff at the London School of Hygiene & Tropical Medicine with considerable experience of teaching public health to students from low, middle and high income countries. Much of the material has been developed and tested with postgraduate students both in face-to-face teaching and through distance learning.

The books are designed for self-directed learning. Each chapter has explicit learning objectives, key terms are highlighted and the text contains many activities to enable the reader to test their own understanding of the ideas and material covered. Written in a clear and accessible style, the series will be essential reading for students taking postgraduate courses in public health and will also be of interest to public health practitioners and policy-makers.

Titles in the series

Analytical models for decision making: Colin Sanderson and Reinhold Gruen
Controlling communicable disease: Norman Noah
Economic analysis for management and policy: Stephen Jan, Lilani Kumaranayake,
    Jenny Roberts, Kara Hanson and Kate Archibald
Economic evaluation: Julia Fox-Rushby and John Cairns (eds)
Environmental epidemiology: Paul Wilkinson (ed)
Environment, health and sustainable development: Megan Landon
Environmental health policy: David Ball (ed)
Financial management in health services: Reinhold Gruen and Anne Howarth
Global change and health: Kelley Lee and Jeff Collin (eds)
Health care evaluation: Sarah Smith, Don Sinclair, Rosalind Raine and Barnaby Reeves
Health promotion practice: Maggie Davies, Wendy Macdowall and Chris Bonell (eds)
Health promotion theory: Maggie Davies and Wendy Macdowall (eds)
Introduction to epidemiology: Lucianne Bailey, Katerina Vardulaki, Julia Langham and
    Daniel Chandramohan
Introduction to health economics: David Wonderling, Reinhold Gruen and Nick Black
Issues in public health: Joceline Pomerleau and Martin McKee (eds)
Making health policy: Kent Buse, Nicholas Mays and Gill Walt
Managing health services: Nick Goodwin, Reinhold Gruen and Valerie Iles
Medical anthropology: Robert Pool and Wenzel Geissler
Principles of social research: Judith Green and John Browne (eds)
Understanding health services: Nick Black and Reinhold Gruen

Health Care Evaluation

Sarah Smith, Don Sinclair, Rosalind Raine and
Barnaby Reeves

Open University Press

Open University Press
McGraw-Hill Education
McGraw-Hill House
Shoppenhangers Road
Maidenhead
Berkshire
England
SL6 2QL

email: enquiries@openup.co.uk
world wide web: www.openup.co.uk

and Two Penn Plaza, New York, NY 10121-2289, USA

First published 2005
Reprinted 2010

A catalogue record of this book is available from the British Library

ISBN-10: 0 335 218490 (pb)
ISBN-13: 978 0 335 218493 (pb)

Library of Congress Cataloging-in-Publication Data
CIP data has been applied for

Typeset by RefineCatch Limited, Bungay, Suffolk
Printed in Great Britain by Ashford Colour Press Ltd, Gosport, Hampshire

Contents

Acknowledgements

Open University Press and the London School of Hygiene & Tropical Medicine have made every effort to obtain permission from copyright holders to reproduce material in this book and to acknowledge these sources correctly. Any omissions brought to our attention will be remedied in future editions.

We would like to express our grateful thanks to the following copyright holders for granting permission to reproduce material in this book.

pp. 78–83   Black N, 'Why we need observational studies to evaluate the effectiveness of health care', *BMJ*, 1996, 312: 1215–1217, reproduced with permission from the BMJ Publishing Group.

pp. 25–26   Donaldson RJ and Donaldson LJ, *Essential Public Health Medicine 2nd edition*, 1993, Radcliffe Publishing. Reprinted by permission of Radcliffe Publishing.

pp. 17–19   Eddy DM, 'Should we change the rules for evaluating medical technologies?' in Gelijins AC (ed), *Modern Methods of clinical investigation.* © 1990. Reprinted with permission from by the National Academy of Sciences, courtesy of the National Academies Press, Washington, DC

pp. 143–146 Fitzpatrick R, 'The assessment of patient satisfaction' in Jenkinson C (ed), *Assessment and evaluation of health and medical care*, 1997, Open University Press.

pp. 30–31   Gosling R, Walraven G, Manneh F, Bailey R, Lewis SM, 'Training health workers to assess anaemia with the WHO haemoglobin colour scale,' *Tropical Medicine and International Health*, 5(3): 214–221, Blackwell Publishing Ltd.

pp. 52–53, 54, 57–58 Grimes DA & Schulz KF, 'Bias and causal associations in observational research'. Reprinted with permission from Elsevier (*The Lancet*, 2002, 359(9302): 248–252).

p. 64   Grimes DA & Schulz KF, 'Allocation concealment in randomised trials: defending against deciphering'. Reprinted with permission from Elsevier (*The Lancet*, 2002, 359(9306): 614–618).

pp. 151–152, 158–159 Layte R and Jenkinson C, 'Social Surveys' in Jenkinson C (ed), *Assessment and evaluation of health and medical care*, 1997, Open University Press.

pp. 94–95   Mant J and Jenkinson C, 'Case control and cohort studies' in Jenkinson C (ed), *Assessment and evaluation of health and medical care*, 1997, Open University Press.

pp. 191–92, 194 Mooney GH, 'Equity in health care: confronting the confusion'. Reprinted from *Effective Health Care*, 1: 179–184, copyright (1983), with permission from Elsevier.

pp. 100–102 Morgenstein H, 'Ecologic studies in epidemiology: Concepts, principles and methods,' *Annual Review of Public Health*, (1995) 16: 61–81. Reprinted by permission of Annual Review.

pp. 40–42   Patrick DL and Deyo RA, Generic and disease-specific measures in assessing health status and quality of life, *Medical Care*, 27: 17–232.

pp. 182–83   Raine R, 'Bias Measuring bias,' *J Health Serv Res Policy* 2002, 7: 65–67 by permission of RSM Publishing.

pp. 67–69   Schulz KF & Grimes DA, 'Sample size slippages in randomised trials: exclusions and the lost and wayward'. Reprinted with permission from Elsevier (*The Lancet*, 2002, 359(9308): 781–785).

p. 98   Sheldon TA et al, 'What's the evidence that NICE guidance has been implemented? Results from a national evaluation using time series analysis, audit of patients' notes, and interviews,' *BMJ*, 2004, 329: 999–1006, reproduced with permission from the BMJ Publishing Group.

pp. 71–73   Shepperd S, Doll H and Jenkinson C, 'Randomised controlled trials' in Jenkinson C (ed), *Assessment and evaluation of health and medical care*, 1997, Open University Press.

pp. 154–56   Stone DH, 'Design a questionnaire,' *BMJ*, 1993, 307: 1264–6, reproduced with permission from the BMJ Publishing Group.

pp. 127–29, 132–135 Watson K, 'Economic evaluation of health care' in Jenkinson C (ed), *Assessment and evaluation of health and medical care*, 1997, Open University Press.

pp. 166–68, 169, 171–172, 173–75 Ziebland S and Wright L, 'Qualitative research methods' in Jenkinson C (ed), *Assessment and evaluation of health and medical care*, 1997, Open University Press.

Overview of the book

Introduction

Throughout the world, health care is practised in a wide variety of ways. Nearly every society seeks improved health for its members. When the basic necessities for survival have been met the search for better health is often pursued by seeking better forms of health care. No nation can afford to provide all the health care that its population would want. It can, however, ensure that it obtains the greatest benefit from those resources available for health care. This is where the systematic evaluation of health care can help.

Why study health care evaluation?

The process of evaluation seeks to analyse health care interventions in terms of four key dimensions: effectiveness, efficiency, humanity and equity. This process can be used to compare one or more interventions in such a way that the policy-makers can choose which to provide for their population. Hence, evaluation is a key activity of health services research. Even if you are not performing evaluative research yourself, as a manager you need to develop an awareness of the methods used and the interpretation of results. Putting health care evaluation into practice is an essential process of health care planning and management.

This book uses a multidisciplinary approach to describe and illustrate the methods available for evaluation of health services. By the end you should be able to describe key methods for evaluating the effectiveness, efficiency, equity and humanity of health care and apply them to specific health care interventions.

Structure of the book

The six sections, and the 17 chapters within them, are shown on the book's contents page. Each chapter includes:

- an overview;
- a list of learning objectives;
- a list of key terms;
- a range of activities;
- feedback on the activities;
- a summary.

Health care and evaluation

The first chapter in this section introduces the idea of health as a multidimensional concept. The material in the chapter explores what is meant by health care, who provides health care and why it is necessary to evaluate health care. The second chapter begins by defining evaluation and introducing the importance of a scientific approach. The chapter also provides an overview of the range of scientific methods (including an overview of randomized studies, non-randomized methods, ecological studies and descriptive methods) and makes the distinction between quantitative and qualitative approaches. This chapter also introduces the four dimensions of effectiveness, efficiency, humanity and equity.

Measuring disease, health status and health-related quality of life

The first chapter in this section describes what is meant by disease measures and reviews the scientific criteria by which all measures should be evaluated. Sources of bias in disease measurement and methods for minimizing them are discussed. Finally the sources of data for measuring disease are described. The second chapter in this section explores the conceptual distinctions between terms such as health status, functional status and health-related quality of life. The rest of the chapter compares generic and disease-specific approaches to measurement and reviews cross-cultural approaches to measurement of health-related quality of life.

Evaluating effectiveness

The first chapter in this section makes the distinctions between effectiveness and efficacy, methods for demonstrating a statistical association and causality. Internal and external validity are also discussed. Subsequent chapters describe randomized methods (Chapter 6), non-randomized methods (including cohort studies and case-control studies) (Chapters 7 and 8) and ecological studies (Chapter 9). The final chapter provides an opportunity to review and compare the study designs covered in previous chapters.

Measuring cost and evaluating cost-effectiveness

The first chapter in this section explains why cost information is important and describes what is meant by recurrent and capital costs, direct, indirect and opportunity costs and intangible costs. The chapter goes on to consider who bears costs, sources of cost information and the stages of measuring cost. The principle of discounting is briefly considered. Chapter 12 describes four types of economic analysis (cost-minimization analysis, cost-effectiveness analysis, cost-benefit analysis and cost-utility analysis). The chapter also describes the steps in performing a cost-effectiveness analysis and the principle of using quality-adjusted life years in a cost-utility analysis.

Evaluating humanity

Chapter 13 introduces four dimensions of humanity (autonomy, dignity, beneficence and non-maleficence). The chapter then reviews the circumstances where
health care can lack humanity and possible limits to humanity. The relationship
between patient satisfaction with the process of health care and humanity is also
discussed. Chapters 14 and 15 respectively review quantitative and qualitative
methods for evaluating humanity.

Evaluating equity

Chapter 16 introduces the concept of equity and describes some of the main ethical
theories (utilitarianism, Kantianism, liberal individualism, communitarian theories, principle-based, common-morality theories). Equity is operationally defined in
terms of horizontal and vertical equity. The final chapter considers the definition
of need and description of what influences need (geographical factors, socioeconomic factors, ethnic factors, age etc.) and ways of assessing need. Definitions
of equity (equality of expenditure per capita, equality of inputs per capita, quality
of input for equal need, equality of access for equal need, equality of utilization
for equal need, equality of marginal met need, equality of health) are also considered as are trade-offs between equity and efficiency and between equity and
effectiveness.

Acknowledgements

The authors acknowledge the important contributions made by colleagues who
developed the original lectures and teaching material at the LSHTM on which some of
the contents are based: Nick Black (Chapters 1, 2, 6–8); Donna Lamping (Chapter 4);
Colin Sanderson (Chapter 9); Charles Normand (Chapters 11 and 12); Rebecca Rosen
(Chapters 13–15). The authors also thank the following for helpful comments: Nick
Black, Donna Lamping, John Cairns, Hannah-Rose Douglas and Andrew Hutchings.
Finally, we thank Steve George at the University of Southampton for reviewing the book
and Deirdre Byrne (project manager) for help and support.

SECTION I

Health care and evaluation

Introduction to health and health care

Overview

This chapter provides a brief introduction to the concepts of health and health care. You will consider a broad definition of health, and why it is not always appropriate to think of ill health simply in terms of disease.

Learning objectives

By the end of this chapter you should be able to:

- **describe the multidimensional nature of the concept of health**
- **outline the range of activities that can be considered as health care**
- **give examples of the different agencies involved in providing health care**
- **explain the need to evaluate health care**

Key terms

Evaluation The critical assessment of the value of an activity.

Health care Any activity that is intended to improve the state of physical, mental or social function of people.

What is health?

In the last few decades there has been a move away from conceptualizing health as simply the absence of illness. More recent definitions have encouraged a more positive and multidimensional concept of health, usually including physical, social and psychological components. The constitution of the World Health Organization (WHO) (1947) provides a basis for thinking about health in broader terms and defines health as 'a state of complete physical, mental and social well-being, and not merely the absence of disease or infirmity'. A fourth component of 'autonomy' has since been added (WHO 1984). The term 'health' can be thought of as an umbrella term that encompasses several other states (e.g. health status, functional status, health-related quality of life, quality of life). These terms are sometimes used interchangeably, though in fact each has a distinct definition. These terms will be discussed in later chapters.

The WHO definition of health also enables us to consider health as a subjective phenomenon. Well-being can mean different things to different people and individuals may therefore perceive the same disease or disability differently. For example, consider someone who lives with a chronic disability. A disability that is stable, such as a congenital limb abnormality, may not be seen as a manifestation of disease by the individual concerned. Appropriate appliances and treatment (such as physiotherapy) may be used to improve the quality of such people's lives and thus contribute to their well-being. Providing help with daily tasks, such as carrying food and water, could also improve well-being (health). Despite its conceptual importance, recognizing that health includes a subjective component also presents some methodological challenges, some of which we will discuss later.

What is health care?

Health care is an activity with a *primary intention* to improve health, as opposed to other activities which have indirect health effects (such as education or housing). Health care comprises a wide spectrum of activities including, for example, health promotion, disease prevention, curative care, rehabilitation, long-term and palliative care. Health care also expands beyond the formal sector into the informal sector, and also includes lay care. The availability of health care from lay people may determine how much health care by professionals is needed. A working definition of health care for the purposes of health care evaluation might be 'any activity that is intended to improve the state of physical, mental or social function for one or more people'.

Who provides health care?

Considering the definitions above, it is clear that there are many different groups of people providing health care. Professional carers (doctors, nurses, physiotherapists, for example) are easily recognized, but throughout the world most health care is performed by lay people. Parents care for sick children. Children care for elderly parents. Many voluntary organizations care for the ill, the homeless and the disabled. In many countries, social services provide care for many groups of people. This care is intended to improve the well-being of the recipients. As such, it may be considered to be health care.

As defined above, health care aims to improve health by improving physical, mental or social well-being. For example, physical well-being might be improved by increasing mobility, mental well-being might be improved by reducing anxiety and social well-being might be improved by enabling people to have more social contacts.

Activity 1.1 will give you the opportunity to think of some examples of health care in each of these three categories.

Activity 1.1

Consider the health care provided in your own community. List some examples of health care that aim to improve:

1 Physical health.
2 Mental health.
3 Social health.

List some of the agencies that are involved in providing these forms of health care.

 Feedback

Here are some examples of the sorts of care provided in communities, and the types of agencies involved.

1 Physical health – preventing illness, by immunization against infectious disease (provided by medical and nursing professionals) or screening (e.g. breast cancer screening for women). Prevention could also be achieved through setting up campaigns against smoking or excess alcohol consumption (provided by various agencies including social services and voluntary organizations). Treatment of disease, such as diarrhoeal illness relieved with oral rehydration (provided by medical and nursing professionals and lay carers).

2 Mental health – staffed hostels enabling people with mental illness to live in the community (provided by social services, often with the support of voluntary agencies and community psychiatric nurses). Treatment of the severely mentally ill with medication (provided by medical and nursing professionals). Prevention of illness by screening new mothers for post-natal depression (provided by nurses).

3 Social health – providing social amenities such as community centres, where people can meet (provided by local authorities and voluntary organizations). Providing leisure centres, where people can meet but that will also have a physical health benefit by encouraging people to participate in exercise (provided by local authorities).

Clearly, many different agencies can be involved in providing health care. Often the delivery of effective care involves different organizations working closely together in partnership to tackle different aspects of the same problem. The example above of caring for the mentally ill within the community involves health care professionals (doctors and nurses) working with social services and a number of voluntary agencies to provide suitable accommodation with supervision of treatment.

What is the purpose of evaluating health care?

Jenkinson (1997) provides a useful summary of evaluation in the context of health care. He argues that evaluation provides evidence for decisions about which services should be provided by identifying which interventions work and which are affordable. Jenkinson goes on to say that the limited resources available for health care mean that evaluation is increasingly important in the planning of health care provision. It is important to match the health care provided to the needs of the population. However, because health care is expensive, it is also necessary to choose those interventions that produce the greatest health gains at the lowest cost. Traditionally, evaluation has often been based on intuition and only a relatively small number of interventions have been evaluated rigorously. The type of health care that is available and its location have therefore been shaped by historical patterns of supply and demand and it has not always been easy for planners to make major changes to the provision of health care.

Summary

In this chapter you have considered health as a broad concept in terms of physical, mental and social well-being. You have seen that health is a subjective concept and that individuals' ideas of health and well-being may vary according to their own circumstances.

Health care has been defined as any activity with a primary intention to improve health. You have seen that there is a broad spectrum of activities that may be regarded as health care. These are performed by a wide range of agencies, including health care professionals and members of social services, voluntary organizations and lay people.

You have considered the need to evaluate health interventions in order to provide those that work, and cease providing those that don't. You have also been introduced to the need to use more detailed evaluation to maximize the benefits of health care within the available resources.

References

Jenkinson C (1997) Assessment and evaluation of health and medical care: an introduction and overview, in Jenkinson C (ed.) *Assessment and evaluation of health and medical care.* Buckingham: Open University Press.

WHO (World Health Organization) (1947) *Constitution of the World Health Organization.* Geneva: WHO.

WHO (World Health Organization) (1984) *Uses of epidemiology in aging: report of a scientific group, 1983*, technical report series no. 706. Geneva: WHO.

2 | Introduction to evaluation

Overview

In Chapter 1, you considered the need to evaluate health care. In this chapter, you will begin to examine the scientific approach to evaluation. This is based upon measuring the extent to which a particular health care intervention meets specified health objectives. This chapter will review what is meant by evaluation and will introduce the dimensions by which health care can be evaluated.

Learning objectives

By the end of this chapter you should be better able to:

- **explain the purpose of evaluation and distinguish between research and audit**
- **describe the four main dimensions of evaluation: effectiveness, efficiency, humanity and equity**
- **outline the steps involved in designing an evaluation**
- **identify the wide range of scientific approaches and study designs that can be used in evaluation**

Key terms

Bias An error that results in a systematic deviation from the estimation of the association between exposure and outcome.

Effectiveness The extent to which an intervention produces a beneficial result under usual conditions of clinical care.

Efficiency (cost-effectiveness) The cost of providing a health care intervention in relation to the improvement of health outcomes.

Equity Fairness, defined in terms of equality of opportunity, provision, use or outcome.

Humanity The quality of being civil, courteous or obliging to others.

What is evaluation?

The process of evaluation seeks to measure how a change in the way that care is provided affects the health of individuals or populations. Usually one form of health care is compared with another or with no care. The term 'health care evaluation' has a specific meaning in the context of health services research (HSR), which can be defined as follows: 'Health care evaluation is the critical assessment on as scientifically rigorous a basis as possible of the degree to which health services fulfil stated objectives'. The first part of this definition places emphasis on the 'scientific' approach, the second on the 'objectives' of health care. We will look at them both in turn.

There is a range of evaluative sciences from basic science to policy, and Table 2.1 illustrates the focus of each and the place HSR occupies in this spectrum. Clearly, there are interrelations and connections between the research fields, but each has its own approach to the subject and makes a distinct contribution to the evaluation of health care. HSR requires input from a large range of disciplines such as medicine, nursing, sociology, economics, epidemiology, statistics and psychology.

Table 2.1 The focus of various forms of research

Disciplinary research	Biomedical research	Clinical research	Health services research	Public health research
Focuses on theory	Focuses on organisms	Focuses on individuals	Focuses on systems	Focuses on communities

The use of evaluation within the research context is distinct from its use within other management activities such as quality assurance and monitoring. These are applicable only to a particular context, whereas research aims to be generalizable across different contexts. As health care is multifaceted and can involve a variety of different agencies, evaluation also needs to be multidisciplinary. Thus the overall judgement of a particular health care requires the outcome to be favourable from each of these perspectives. The chapters that follow will discuss in more detail how each of these disciplines contributes to effective evaluation.

The range of scientific methods

The variety of methods that have been used in evaluation can be described as a spectrum, from simple intuition to rigorous science (Hammond and Arkes 1986). Scientific methods, including both quantitative and qualitative techniques, aim to provide high quality evidence that minimizes bias and confounding factors. However, there can sometimes be a trade-off between the quality of the scientific evidence and the time and resources required to obtain it.

All methods have strengths and weaknesses and also vary in the extent to which they are able to eliminate bias (or systematic error) and confounding. When they are feasible and appropriate, randomized controlled trials (RCTs) provide strong quantitative evidence for use in evaluation. The RCT is now often upheld as the 'gold standard' method for obtaining rigorous, scientific evidence. There are also situations where an RCT is unnecessary, inappropriate, impossible or inadequate (Black 1996). In these situations observational methods such as non-randomized trials, retrospective and prospective cohort studies, case-control and ecological studies provide alternative or complementary evidence. All of these methods can be used for evaluation. However each investigator has to ensure that the study is designed properly, the variables are measured accurately and reliably and the findings are interpreted appropriately.

Qualitative methods can also be used in evaluation. These tend to address questions such as 'How?' and 'Why?' whereas quantitative methods are more useful for answering questions such as 'How much?' or 'How often?'. For both types of method data collection and analysis can be based on either individuals or groups. Often there may be a choice of study designs to answer the same question.

Defining objectives

Health interventions should be evaluated in terms of their ability to fulfil specific objectives. Objectives are statements of what an intervention is supposed to do. These should be measurable and specified as precisely as possible. For any evaluation the objectives are assessed by measuring the outcomes of the intervention. The exact nature of the outcomes will depend on the nature of the intervention. However, simply knowing how an outcome changed as a result of the intervention would not be sufficient to evaluate the service. Some specific standards are needed in order to assess health care outcomes. These are discussed below in terms of four dimensions for evaluation.

Activity 2.1 will give you an opportunity to specify the objectives for a form of health care and consider how you might measure whether they have been achieved.

 Activity 2.1

Imagine a health care intervention with which you are familiar. A day centre for the mentally ill or cardiac transplantation for cardiomyopathy are examples, but it could be anything at all. Specify as precisely as possible the objectives that this intervention aims to achieve, and that you would evaluate. Next consider how you would measure whether the intervention actually achieves these stated objectives.

 Feedback

Using as an example the evaluation of a new day centre for patients suffering from mental illness, here are examples of both a poor and a good statement of objectives.

a) *A poor statement of objectives:* '. . . to determine the effectiveness of a day centre for patients with mental illness'.

b) *A good statement of objectives:* '. . . to determine whether patients suffering from moderate depression require fewer admissions to psychiatric hospitals if they are offered twice-weekly attendance at a day centre'.

As part of the definition of this evaluation, it would be necessary to define moderate depression. For example, using a standard diagnostic questionnaire would enable you to be explicit about what was meant by moderate depression, particularly if the diagnostic tool had well-established cut-off points. The nature of the psychiatric day centre would also need to be defined. This could be described in terms of the type of staff (e.g. the balance of medical or nursing staff to lay staff) and the type of activities in which patients can participate.

Possible outcomes might include:

- the proportion of patients offered twice-weekly attendance at the day centre, who subsequently require admission to psychiatric hospital
- the mean number of psychiatric admissions for patients attending the day centre
- the reasons why patients who attend the day centre require fewer psychiatric admissions

The first two require quantitative evidence and would enable comparison with other similar centres or change over time. More qualitative methods could be used to assess reasons why day centre attendance reduces psychiatric admissions.

The four dimensions of health care evaluation

Health care interventions are usually evaluated in terms of effectiveness, efficiency (which is often referred to as cost-effectiveness), humanity and equity.

- *Effectiveness* describes the benefits of health services measured by improvements in health in a real population. Sometimes publications describe the benefits of health care in terms of efficacy. Efficacy describes the benefits obtainable from an intervention under ideal conditions, such as in a specialist centre. The evaluation of effectiveness is considered in detail in Chapters 5–10.
- *Efficiency* (or cost-effectiveness) relates the cost of an intervention to the benefits obtained. Ideally the benefits should be measured in terms of the degree of health gained. This is sometimes difficult to achieve. Cost and cost-effectiveness are discussed in Chapters 11 and 12. There are however other definitions of efficiency. In particular, governments sometimes use the term 'efficiency' to refer to increased *productivity*. This is somewhat confusing, but throughout this book we will use the term 'efficiency' to refer to *cost-effectiveness* rather than increased productivity.
- *Humanity* is the quality of being humane. It describes the social, psychological and ethical acceptability of the treatment that people receive from a health care intervention. In some situations, such as the forced restraint of patients, it may be obvious that treatment is inhumane. In other situations it may be less clear. Humanity is considered in detail in Chapters 13 and 15.
- *Equity* refers to the fair distribution of health services among groups or individuals. One cause of inequity may be that some groups (frequently the poor) are less able to access health services than others. The evaluation of equity is considered in Chapters 16 and 17.

Whether an intervention is appropriate for a population or individual is related to these four dimensions. If an intervention is not appropriate, it may either be because it is less effective or more expensive than an alternative, or because it is simply not acceptable, perhaps for cultural reasons or because it is not available for certain groups of people. In practice, interventions are rarely perfect in all dimensions. Interpreting the results of evaluation therefore often involves hard choices in trading one dimension against another.

When a new intervention is introduced, it should be evaluated in terms of effectiveness, cost-effectiveness (or efficiency), humanity and equity. However, for an established intervention it may only be necessary to evaluate the dimensions for which there is uncertainty about the outcome. For both new and established interventions, it is always necessary to be explicit about which dimensions are to be considered in a particular evaluation.

Activity 2.2 provides an opportunity to think about an example of a health intervention in terms of these four dimensions.

 Activity 2.2

Consider a plan to introduce a new childhood immunization programme against measles. Assume that, in this example, children are to be immunized at the ages of 13 months and 4 years. Suppose that you have been asked by the Ministry of Health to evaluate this service. Write down the objectives of the service that you would evaluate. Under the headings of effectiveness, efficiency, humanity and equity, list the information that you would require to evaluate each of these dimensions for the service.

 Feedback

Your answer should include points similar to the following.

Objectives
- to achieve a reduction in the incidence of cases of measles in the target population
- to achieve a reduction in the incidence of deaths from measles in the target population

Effectiveness
The outcome of interest could be vaccine efficacy (measured as the proportion of children immunized who became resistant to measles). You would also be interested in the reduction in incidence of cases of (or deaths from) measles in the target population that are attributable to immunization. This would be assessed by calculating the incidence before and some years after the introduction of the immunization programme – assuming that any change in incidence can be attributed fully to the programme itself.

Efficiency
The outcomes of interest could be cost per case of measles prevented and cost per death from measles prevented. These should be measured in terms of monetary costs, of the vaccine but should also include the cost of transport to attend clinics, and the loss of earnings if time must be taken from work to attend.

Humanity
The outcome of interest would be acceptability of immunization to parents and children. This will be influenced by local culture and the perception of measles as an important problem in the target population. Qualitative interviews with both parents

who chose to immunize their children and those whose children were not immunized could help to determine why immunization was acceptable to some, but not to others.

Equity
All elements of the population should be equally represented among those who accept immunization. Even if the vaccination is free, travel cost may deter poorer families. If immunization is perceived as beneficial but resources are limited, there may be preference for immunization of one sex rather than the other. Equity could be assessed by comparing the rates of immunization of children from different socioeconomic backgrounds.

Perspectives in evaluation

The emphasis given to different dimensions may depend on the perspective from which the evaluation is viewed. For example, the approach taken may differ according to whether you take the viewpoint of a health district or of central government as a whole. In the activity you have just completed you were asked to take the perspective of the Ministry of Health. In this case emphasis might be placed on cost-effectiveness (efficiency), particularly if health care is funded centrally. In contrast, a local health district might place more emphasis on dimensions that impact on the local community. For example, if uptake of the vaccine was particularly low, the local health district might place more emphasis on the reasons why immunisation is acceptable to some but not others.

Steps in designing an evaluation

1 Describe the objectives of your evaluation. These need to be precise, and should contain a description of the intervention or interventions that will be evaluated and the population who will receive them.
2 Choose which of the four dimensions (effectiveness, efficiency, humanity and equity) are to be evaluated. This will depend on the nature of the health care intervention and the perspective from which the evaluation will be undertaken.
3 Determine which outcome measures can be used to assess the chosen dimensions for these interventions.
4 Choose a study design which is able to evaluate the chosen dimensions.
5 Identify appropriate data sources and plan how and when to collect data.

In later chapters you will consider in detail the appropriate types of study to use for evaluating each dimension.

Bias and confounders

The article below by Eddy (1990) describes some of the different types of bias that can affect particular study designs. Bias indicates a systematic error and all good research aims to minimize bias. Bias occurs when data relating to one group of patients are systematically different from the data relating to the other groups of patients. This means that any difference in measured outcomes between the groups may be due to bias and not to the different technologies used. A confounder is a characteristic that is an independent risk factor for the outcome under study as well as being associated with the intervention. If the sources of confounding can be anticipated, its effects can be controlled. There are many different forms of bias and these and more detail about confounding will be described in more detail in the chapters that describe ways of evaluating effectiveness (Chapters 5–9).

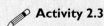

Activity 2.3

Read the extract below and then answer the following questions:

1 What are the four criteria that a new technology must satisfy before it should be introduced?
2 What is meant by internal validity?
3 What is meant by external validity?
4 Why are results from certain studies more credible than those from others?

Should we change the rules for evaluating the effectiveness of health care

Before we launch a new medical technology, we would like to show that it satisfies four criteria:
– It improves the health outcomes patients care about: pain, death, anxiety, disfigurement, disability.
– Its benefits outweigh its harms.
– Its health effects are worth its costs.
– And, if resources are limited, it deserves priority over other technologies.

To apply any of these criteria we need to estimate the magnitude of the technology's benefits and harms. We want to gather this information as accurately, quickly, and inexpensively as possible to speed the use of technologies that have these properties and direct our energy away from technologies that do not.

There are many ways to estimate a technology's benefits and harms. They range from simply asking experts (pure clinical judgment) to conducting multiple randomized controlled trials, with anecdotes, clinical series, data bases, non-randomized controlled trials, and case-control studies in between. The choice of a method has great influence on the cost of the evaluation, the duration of time required for the evaluation, the accuracy of the information gained, the complexity of administering the evaluation, and the ease of defending the subsequent decisions.

The problem before us is to determine which set of methods delivers information of sufficiently high quality to draw conclusions with confidence, at the lowest cost in time and money . . .

Biases

. . . It is convenient to separate biases into two types. Biases to internal validity affect the accuracy of the results of the study as an estimate of the effect of the technology in the setting in which a study was conducted (e.g., the specific technology, specific patient indications, and so forth). Biases to external validity affect the applicability of the results to other settings (where the techniques, patient indications, and other factors might be different).

Examples of biases to internal validity include patient selection bias, crossover, errors in measurement of outcomes, and errors in ascertainment of exposure to the technology. Patient selection bias exists when patients in the two groups to be compared (e.g., the control and treated groups of a controlled trial) differ in ways that could affect the outcome of interest. When such differences exist, a difference in outcomes could be due at least in part to inherent differences in the patients, not to the technology. Crossover occurs either when patients in the group offered the technology do not receive it (sometimes called 'dilution') or when patients in the control group get the technology (sometimes called 'contamination'). Errors in measurement of outcomes can affect a study's results if the technique used to measure outcomes (e.g., claims data, patient interviews, urine tests, blood samples) do not accurately measure the true outcome. Patients can be misclassified as having had the outcome of interest (e.g., death from breast cancer) when in fact they did not, and vice versa. Errors in ascertainment of exposure to the technology can have an effect similar to crossover. A crucial step in a retrospective study is to determine who got the technology of interest and who did not. These measurements frequently rely on old records and fallible memories. Any errors affect the results.

An example of bias to external validity is the existence of differences between the people studied in the experiment and the people about whom you want to draw conclusions (sometimes called a 'population bias'). For example, they might be older or sicker. Another example occurs when the technology used in the experiment differs from the technology of interest, because of differences in technique, equipment, provider skill, or changes in the technology since the experiment was performed. This is sometimes called 'intensity bias'.

Different evaluative methods are vulnerable to different biases. At the risk of gross oversimplification, Table 2.2 illustrates the vulnerabilities of different designs to biases.

Table 2.2 Susceptibility of various designs to biases

| Design | Internal validity | | | | External validity | |
	Patient selection	Crossover	Error in measurement of outcomes	Error in ascertainment of exposure	Population	Technology
RCT	0	++	+	0	++	++
Non-RCT	+	+	+	0	+	+
CCS	++	0	+	+++	0	0
Comparison of clinical series	+++	0	+	0	+	+
Data bases	++	0	++	++	0	0

0 implies minimal vulnerability to a bias.
+++ implies high vulnerability to a bias.
RCT, randomized controlled trials; CCS, case-control studies.

A zero implies that the bias is either nonexistent or likely to be negligible; three plus signs indicate that the bias is likely to be present and to have an important effect on the observed outcome. Methodologists can debate my choices, and there are innumerable conditions and subtle issues that will prevent agreement from ever being reached; the point is not to produce a definitive table of biases, but to convey the general message that all the designs are affected by biases, and the patterns are different for different designs.

For example, a major strength of the randomized controlled trial is that it is virtually free of patient selection biases. Indeed, that is the very purpose of randomization. In contrast, non-randomized controlled trials, case-control studies, and data bases are all subject to patient selection biases. On the other hand, randomized controlled trials are more affected by crossover than the other three designs. All studies are potentially affected by errors in measurement of outcomes, with data bases more vulnerable than most because they are limited to whatever data elements were originally chosen by the designers. Case-control studies are especially vulnerable to mis-specification of exposure to the technology, because of their retrospective nature. Data bases can be subject to the same problem, depending on the accuracy with which the data elements were coded.

With respect to external validity, randomized controlled trials are sensitive to population biases, because the recruitment process and admission criteria often result in a narrowly defined set of patient indications. Randomized controlled trials are also vulnerable to concerns that the intensity and quality of care might be different in research settings than in actual practice. The distinction between the 'efficacy' of a technology (in research settings) and the 'effectiveness' of a technology (in routine practice) reflects this concern. Thus, the results of a trial might not be widely applicable to other patient indications or less controlled settings. Data bases and case-control studies, on the other hand, tend to draw from 'real' populations. All designs are susceptible to changes in the technology but in different ways. Because they are prospective, randomized controlled trials and non-randomized controlled trials are vulnerable to future changes. Because they are retrospective, case-control studies and retrospective analyses of data bases are vulnerable to differences between the present and the past.

 Feedback

1 Before introducing a new technology, it should be shown to:

   a) improve the health outcomes that actually matter to patients
   b) produce a greater amount of benefit than harm
   c) produce health benefits that are worth the cost incurred
   d) deserve priority over other technologies competing for the same resources.

2 Internal validity describes how well a study measures the effects of a technology in the circumstances of the study. In other words, it describes how well the study measures efficacy, because it relates to the population taking part in the study and to the circumstances of care that they receive.

3 External validity describes how well the effects of a technology measured in a study can be expected to apply to patients outside the study environment. If the study population is highly selected it may not represent those who will actually need the technology in the wider community. You would be unlikely to achieve the same degree of effectiveness as measured in the study.

4 The extract does not provide an exhaustive list of all types of bias, but does provide examples of some of the types of bias that can occur in particular studies. The important point is that all study designs are potentially affected by bias and that different types of

study are subject to different types of bias. This is one reason why different types of study are appropriate to answer different questions. The table in the article provides a summary of the way that different biases affect different types of study. Do not spend too long trying to learn these now. You will consider them in more detail with possible solutions in later chapters. In general, RCTs tend to have less bias relating to allocation of patients (as they are randomized), but may have bias related to 'crossover' (where patients switch treatment part way through a study). The narrow inclusion criteria often used in RCTs may also mean that the results are not generalizable to the population from which the sample was drawn. Non-randomized studies are more prone to allocation bias, though less likely to have problems relating to crossover bias. Non-randomized studies are also less likely to have biases relating to generalizability. Bias or error relating to the measurement of outcomes is likely to occur in both randomized and non-randomized studies. In general biases such as 'dilution' and 'contamination' are less problematic than other biases which might result in exaggeration of a treatment effect.

Summary

In this chapter you have seen how health care is provided to meet specific objectives. When evaluating health care, these objectives must be stated as precisely as possible. You have considered the four dimensions of health care evaluation (effectiveness, cost-effectiveness, humanity and equity) and how they would be relevant to evaluating one example of health care (measles immunization).

New interventions should be evaluated in terms of all four dimensions. When comparing alternative established interventions, it may only be necessary to measure those dimensions that are likely to show differences between the interventions.

You have learned that the purpose of an evaluation may vary according to the perspective taken, and how this can affect the emphasis applied to different dimensions.

References

Black NA (1996) Why we need observational studies to evaluate the effectiveness of health care. *British Medical Journal* 312: 1215–18.
Eddy DM (1990) Should we change the rules for evaluating medical technologies? in Gelijns AC (ed.) *Modern methods of clinical investigation*. Washington, DC: National Academy Press.
Hammond K R and Arkes H (1986) Judgment and Decision Making: an interdisciplinary reader. Boulder Colorado, Westview Press, pp11–32.

SECTION 2

Measuring disease, health status and health-related quality of life

3 | Measuring disease

Overview

In this chapter you will consider why and how to measure disease and the scientific criteria by which such measures should be evaluated. You will learn about the possible biases that can affect disease measurement and how disease measures can be used to adjust for confounding factors. You will also consider the advantages and disadvantages of a range of sources of data for measuring disease.

Learning objectives

By the end of this chapter you should be able to:

- critically appraise a range of measures of disease and describe their appropriate use in health care evaluation
- describe the scientific criteria for evaluating measures
- identify potential sources of bias in measuring disease and ways that it can be prevented
- explain the principle of case-mix and how it affects the relationship between intervention and outcome
- outline the advantages and disadvantages of routine, ad hoc and standardized data

Key terms

Case-mix The mix of cases (or patients) that a provider cares for.

Construct The hypothetical concept that a questionnaire or other type of instrument is intended to measure.

Impairment The physical signs of the condition (pathology), usually measured by clinicians.

Reliability The extent to which an instrument produces consistent results.

Responsiveness The extent to which an instrument detects real changes in the state of health of a person.

Validity The extent to which an instrument measures what it intends to measure.

What is disease measurement?

The concept of disease reflects a combination of physiological characteristics, a person's perception, professional assessment and cultural norms. The WHO (1980) developed a threefold classification of 'impairment', 'disability' and 'handicap'. These three ideas are distinct but conceptually linked. Impairment refers to the disease itself, for example deafness. Disability describes any restriction in activity that results from the impairment. For example, for a deaf person the disability would be an inability to hear. The term handicap describes the consequences of the disability. For example, for a deaf person the resulting handicap might be difficulty in social interaction. This has since been replaced with a new classification that refers to 'impairment' and 'activity limitation' rather than disability, and 'participation restrictions' rather than handicap (WHO 2001). In this chapter we will focus on measures that assess aspects of impairment. Measurement of aspects of health that could broadly be described as activity limitation (disability) and participation restrictions (handicap) will be considered in Chapter 4.

How is disease measurement used in evaluation?

Measures of disease can be used either as outcome measures or as ways of controlling for risk or confounding factors that might distort the main outcome results. Confounding was briefly described in Chapter 2 (and will be discussed in more detail in Chapter 5) and refers to an independent risk factor for both the intervention and the outcome. If a source of confounding can be anticipated in advance then it can be measured and its effects can be controlled. Whether a particular instrument is used as an outcome measure or to measure confounding factors depends on the context rather than the measure itself. Most instruments can be used as either outcomes or to assess confounding factors. It is important that the choice of measure is appropriate for the purpose and that all aspects of disease are measured using standardized instruments. Some applications of disease measures, such as calculating mortality and morbidity, use standard medical diagnostic criteria (e.g. the International Statistical Classification of Diseases and Related Conditions (ICD)) that are applied by a clinician. Other aspects of disease measurement are obtained directly (e.g. blood pressure measures). Many aspects of disease are measured using standardized questionnaires. These can be self-reported by the patient, observer-rated by a clinician or proxy-reported (e.g. when a parent reports on behalf of a child). The accepted standards for judging all measurement methods are described in the next section.

Disease measures as outcomes

In most evaluation studies, outcomes are compared between patients receiving the new treatment and patients receiving the standard treatment. Any difference between the groups would be assumed to represent a difference in the effectiveness of the two treatments. In other words, the measured difference in outcomes could be said to be associated with the difference in treatments. Mortality (the number of deaths caused by the disease) and morbidity (the number of people affected by the disease) are sometimes used as outcomes when it is the impact of the disease on the population rather than the individual that is being assessed. Assessing morbidity, rather than simply the number of people that die, provides richer information about the burden of the disease. Activity 3.1 will introduce you to some of the terms that are important in using mortality and morbidity to assess the burden of disease. Other ways in which disease measures could be used as outcomes include measurement of signs (e.g. blood pressure, temperature, X-rays) and symptoms (e.g. disease-specific checklists or measures of pain). Measures of disease could also be used to assess effects that are the result of the treatment but are not the intended positive effect (e.g. McGill Pain Questionnaire, Melzack and Torgerson 1971; Melzack 1975, 1987). These effects are known as adverse effects or complications.

Activity 3.1

When describing the impact of illness on a population (rather than on an individual), it is usual to refer to the prevalence or incidence of this illness within the population. Read the following extract from an article by Donaldson and Donaldson (1994) that reviews the concepts of point prevalence, period prevalence and incidence. How would you define.

- point prevalence
- period prevalence
- incidence

Prevalence and incidence

 There are two types of measure of illness or morbidity. They are incidence and prevalence. It is important to be able to distinguish between them (Table 3.1).

Incidence and prevalence

The incidence rate measures the number of new cases of a particular disease arising in a population at risk in a certain time period. In contrast, prevalence measures all cases of the disease existing at a point in time (point prevalence) or over a period in time (period prevalence). Although one often speaks of the prevalence rate of a particular disease, strictly speaking it is not correct to refer to prevalence as a rate. More correctly it is a ratio, since it is a static measure and does not incorporate the idea of cases arising through time. The point prevalence measure is often compared to a snapshot of the population. It states the position at a single point in time. In measuring a particular disease, prevalence counts individuals within the whole spectrum of that disease from people who have newly developed the disease to those in its terminal phases; whereas incidence just counts new

Table 3.1 Measures of morbidity

- Incidence: The number of new cases of a disease occurring per unit of population per unit time
- Point prevalence: The number of people with a disease in a defined population at a point in time
- Period prevalence: The number of people with a disease in a defined population over a period of time.

Source: Donaldson and Donaldson (1994)

cases. Thus, prevalence results from two factors: the size of the previous incidence (occurrence of new cases of the disease) and the duration of the condition from its onset to its conclusion (either as recovery or death). In most chronic diseases complete recovery does not occur. Many people develop diseases (for example, chronic bronchitis, peripheral vascular disease, stroke) in middle age which they may carry until their death. The incidence of a condition is an estimate of the risk of developing the disease and hence is of value mainly to those concerned with searching for the causes or determinants of the disease. Knowledge of the prevalence of a condition is of particular value in planning health services or workload, since it indicates the amount of illness requiring care. Relatively uncommon conditions (i.e. those with a low incidence) may become important health problems if people with the disease are kept alive for a long period of time (producing a relatively high prevalence figure). An example of such a condition is chronic renal failure which is rare, yet because dialysis and transplantation can keep sufferers alive, it becomes an important health problem which consumes considerable resources.

 Feedback

Prevalence describes the number of cases of a specific disease existing within the population at one point in time (point prevalence) or over a specified period of time (period prevalence). It is expressed as a ratio, such as 12 cases per 100,000 population. The prevalence depends on the number of new cases diagnosed, the number of cases dying or recovering and the average duration of illness. Incidence describes the number of new cases of a specific disease arising in a particular population over a specified period of time. It is expressed as a rate, such as 12 cases per 100,000 per year.

Disease measures as confounders

Some disease measures can also be used to control for additional factors that may distort the results of the main outcome. Such effects could occur if one group of patients were more seriously ill than the other. This would be described as a difference in 'case-mix'. Case-mix refers to differences between patients in the two treatment groups in terms of factors such as co-morbidity and severity of illness, and also age. Co-morbidity describes any additional disease (other than the one under investigation) that could affect the outcome measure. The best known and most frequently used measure of co-morbidity is the Charlson Index (Charlson *et al.* 1987). Co-morbidity could also be assessed using the Index of Coexistent Disease (Greenfield *et al.* 1993). This scale additionally allows assessment of the degree of severity of each coexistent disease. In general, severity is a measure of how much the patient is affected by the disease under investigation and its complications. Measures of severity are usually disease-specific, but an example of a commonly used instrument for assessing severity of heart disease is the New York Heart Association Classification (Criteria Committee of the New York Heart Association 1964). Age is also important for assessing case-mix as it affects the prognosis for many diseases.

Case-mix is said to 'confound' the association between the treatment and the outcome measure. It may appear to produce associations that do not really exist and can obscure genuine associations. Confounding can occur for many other reasons too. For example, if the new treatment were administered in a well-staffed coronary care unit and compared with standard treatment on a general medical ward, any improvement in survival might really be due to differences in the expertise of nursing care.

Activity 3.2

Suppose that you have been asked to evaluate the effectiveness of a new treatment for patients suffering from acute myocardial infarction (heart attack). Write down the disease outcomes that you would use and some examples of how you would measure them. The key to this activity lies in thinking what might happen to a patient who has suffered from a heart attack.

Feedback

You could have included such outcomes as:

- death – could be recorded as the proportion of myocardial infarction patients dying within a specified time after admission
- further myocardial infarction (reinfarction) – could be measured as the proportion of patients suffering another myocardial infarction following discharge
- angina (chest pain of varying severity) – could be measured in terms of exercise tolerance, frequency of chest pain events per week or using a standardized pain instrument administered before and after the treatment
- heart failure – could be measured as the proportion of patients who experienced heart failure after the treatment (using ICD criteria)
- recovery (full or partial) – could be measured using standardized functional ability or health status instrument administered before and after the treatment

Note that you could also measure co-morbidity (using for example, the Charlson Index or the Index of Co-existent Disease) to establish whether the group receiving the new treatment had a similar amount of co-existent disease as the group receiving the standard treatment. This would measure a possible confounding factor rather than an outcome and would be used to adjust for case-mix.

Scientific criteria for evaluating measures of disease

There are internationally accepted criteria for judging questionnaire-based measures (Lohr *et al.* 1996; McDowell and Jenkinson 1996; Fitzpatrick *et al.* 1998; Scientific Advisory Committee of the Medical Outcomes Trust 2002). These are sometimes referred to as 'psychometric' criteria. The principles of reliability and validity also apply to measures of disease that are not questionnaire-based (e.g. X-rays). These concepts are described in more detail below. In addition, any alternative forms of the questionnaire, including cross-cultural adaptations, should also meet these standards. Cross-cultural adaptations, should also have linguistic and conceptual equivalence. Respondent burden (the time and effort to complete and/

or administer the instrument) should be minimized in all instruments. These criteria also apply to the measures of health status and health-related quality of life described in Chapter 4.

Reliability is the extent to which the instrument is free from random error. There are several types of reliability (internal consistency, test-retest reliability and inter-rater reliability). As the various type of reliability describe slightly different things, as many types of reliability as are relevant should be assessed. *Test-retest reliability* describes the extent to which the instrument is stable over time, assuming there has been no intervention. It is evaluated using an intra-class correlation. *Internal consistency* describes the extent to which all the items (or questions) in the instrument reflect the same underlying concept (i.e. they are homogenous). It is evaluated using a statistic known as Cronbach's alpha. If the measure is interviewer- or clinician-rated, then *inter-rater reliability* should also be considered. This assesses the extent to which the instrument is stable across different raters. It is assessed by comparing the independent assessment made by two raters, of the same patient, at the same time. Inter-rater reliability is evaluated using an intra-class correlation or a kappa statistic.

Validity describes the extent to which the instrument measures what it purports to measure. There is no single number that represents validity and all the relevant forms of validity should be assessed for a particular instrument. *Content validity* refers to the extent to which all the different aspects of the construct are represented in the instrument. It is assessed by comparing the questions in the instrument with other similar instruments and the existing literature and by consulting with experts. All questionnaires should be based on an explicit conceptual framework and this will also inform content validity. *Criterion-related validity* describes the extent to which a measure is associated with a gold-standard measure of the same construct. In practice it is sometimes difficult to identify a gold standard measure, as the need for a new measure suggests there is not an adequate existing gold standard. *Construct validity* describes the process of investigating whether the measure supports *a priori* hypotheses about relationships between the new instrument and other existing instruments. The new instrument would be expected to be highly related to other instruments measuring the same construct, not related (or low association) with instruments measuring different constructs. Construct validity can also be evaluated by considering the extent to which the new instrument shows the expected difference between two known groups (e.g. a clinical group compared with a control group). Evaluation of construct validity requires an understanding of the construct that is being measured based on the existing literature.

Responsiveness describes the extent to which an instrument can detect clinically meaningful change over time. It can be assessed using a variety of statistics including t-tests (Deyo *et al.* 1991), effect sizes (Cohen 1977; Kazis *et al.* 1990) and standardized response means (Liang *et al.* 1990).

Sources of bias in measures of disease

The reliability and validity of measures of disease can be threatened by a number of factors. These may reflect the way that the instrument was developed, the characteristics of the population under investigation or the way that the instrument was used. All of these factors must be considered for a measurement to be accurate.

We have already discussed the importance of reliability, validity and responsiveness for ensuring good measurement of disease. However, these properties are not always rigorously assessed and there are several frequently-used measures for which there is little evidence of reliability and validity. For example, the New York Heart Association Classification is widely used as an outcome measure in clinical trials, but has little evidence to support its reliability or validity (see Bowling 1997, 2001 for a review of the psychometric properties of this and a variety of other measures). It is the responsibility of each investigator to choose appropriate and robust measures that have adequate reliability and validity.

Strong reliability and validity are equally important for non-questionnaire measures. For example, X-rays, oxygenation saturation or blood pressure all need to be assessed to ensure that they are measuring in a way that is reliable and valid. This means that the necessary equipment must be designed, constructed and calibrated properly. However, in clinical measures such as these, interpretation must also be conducted in a reliable way. For example, there are several classification systems that are used for interpretation of X-rays. For the X-ray to be valid and reliable, these must be used consistently by the clinicians examining the films. There is evidence to suggest that inter-observer agreement (inter-rater reliability) for evaluation of X-rays is relatively low (McCaskie *et al.* 1996). In this example, explicit, standardized criteria would help ensure reliability of X-ray interpretation.

The reliability and validity of even a basic clinical measurement such as height can be threatened by a lack of explicit criteria and instructions. A study to evaluate antenatal clinics in four African countries (Benin, Congo, Senegal and Zaire) where all mothers who were less than 150cm tall were recommended to deliver at home, found that the distribution of maternal height was bi-modal with a peak at 150cm and another at 160cm (in an unselected population, height would be expected to be normally distributed) (Dujardin *et al.* 1993). Despite training instructions, staff were tending to round the measurements (e.g. 150, 155, 160cm) and during busy periods measurement was not being conducted at all, and a 'standard' height was assigned. In addition, on investigation it was discovered that there were strong cultural reasons why first-born children should be delivered at home and also that travel expenses to the hospital from rural areas were prohibitive. It is therefore necessary to monitor all measurements and to re-evaluate them at regular intervals to prevent bias.

Bias can also be introduced to measurement by using an inappropriate person to report the data. There are some occasions when it is necessary to ask a proxy rather than the patient themselves. For example, the patient may be a child who is too young to report for themselves or may have a condition which makes it difficult for them to self-report reliably (e.g. a patient with dementia). Provided that the proxy knows the patient well and is qualified to report on their behalf this is appropriate. Clinician ratings are also routinely used for some measures. For example, to provide joint counts indicating pain in rheumatoid arthritis. This may involve a mannequin picture indicating joints or text, but both methods involve the clinician indicating which joints have pain or tenderness. In a study to compare clinician ratings with self-administered ratings, Calvo *et al.* (1999) found that although both methods were reliable, patients rated pain significantly higher than clinicians. The investigators suggested several possible explanations including the possibility that patients used a different definition of pain that reflected their overall pain experience. They concluded that self-ratings could not be substituted for clinician ratings and that further evidence was needed to compare both types of ratings with evidence from imaging techniques to determine whether ratings are based on structural changes or ongoing inflammation within the joints.

Activity 3.3

Read the following extract from an article by Gosling *et al.* (2000) about haemoglobin assessment. H describes an attempt to train health care workers in a remote area to use the WHO Haemoglobin Colour Scale and the standard WHO training protocol. Once you have read the article, consider the following questions:

1 How could reliability and validity have been threatened by trying to use the Haemoglobin Colour Scale in this area?
2 How were reliability and validity improved?

Training health workers to assess anaemia

Twenty people participated in the study, i.e. 13 Community Health Nurses (CHNs) working at Maternal and Child Health (MCH) clinics in a rural district (Farafenni) and 7 laboratory technicians from the Medical Research Council (MRC) Laboratories, Fajara, The Gambia. CHNs are primary health care workers with a two-year basic training. Part of their job is to run MCH clinics at health facilities including outreach clinics to remote villages. At these clinics pregnant women and all children under five years of age are reviewed. The laboratory technicians had received basic laboratory training and varied considerably in their experience, some were new to the work and others had many years of practice.

The two groups were trained separately four weeks apart. Initially, the training sessions as per the WHO protocol were planned to take place for two hours on each of two consecutive days. This was possible at the MRC Laboratories, but at Farafenni we had to complete both training sessions on one day as the CHNs had to attend a different meeting and had to travel long distances to get to the training centre. Furthermore, the requirement to practice with a set of control bloods was found to be impractical. Despite the resources available for the training at the MRC we were able to obtain only 6 control bloods measuring 15.5, 13.3, 10.0, 8.6, 6.8 and 4.5 g/dl, while for the CHN training we had only 11 control bloods with haemoglobins of 15.7, 14.2, 13.0, 12.2, 11.7, 9.8, 8.3, 6.1, 4.9, 4.5 and 2.7 g/dl. The haemoglobin measurements on these 'reference' samples were obtained using a Celloscope 1260 Analyser (Analysis Instruments AB, Bromma Sweden) at the MRC Laboratories, Fajara, The Gambia which is a participant in the WHO International External Quality Assessment Scheme. No other routine blood samples were available. Accordingly, the training was restructured as follows.

The sessions started with a basic introduction on why the Colour Scale has been developed and its potential use followed by reading through the instructions for use. To overcome difficulty in comprehending the instructions, a cartoon version was prepared . . . which was found to be an excellent complement to the written document.

The technique was demonstrated with a sample of blood of known haemoglobin. The trainees were then asked to test 6 samples of blood (A to F) and to record their haemoglobin estimations. The results were collated on a blackboard and the true haemoglobins (measured by a haemoglobinometer) were revealed. If investigators had a problem with a particular sample they retested that sample under guidance of the instructor until both were satisfied with the result. For training sessions 1 and 2 at the MRC the same samples were used although they were labelled differently for each session. At Farafenni, we split the 11 samples using 5 in the morning and 7 in the afternoon (two samples were used in both sessions.) The training sessions lasted approximately 1.5 h and were held in a well-lit (mixed natural and artificial light) laboratory teaching room at the MRC and in a naturally lit seminar room at Farafenni. At the end of each training session there was a short discussion about the training sessions and how they could be improved.

The CHNs at Farafenni then used the scale to estimate haemoglobin concentrations in women attending their antenatal clinics for a period of one month. They routinely estimated haemoglobins of the women on their first attendance to the clinic and again in the last trimester of pregnancy. The CHNs kept record of their haemoglobin estimations and how they managed the patients, and at the end of the study period completed a qualitative questionnaire about what they thought of the Colour Scale and how it compared to the Buffalo Medical Sciences (BMS) portable haemoglobinometer that they used previously.

 Feedback

1 The authors found that the standard WHO training protocol was not feasible in a remote area where resources were scarce for two main reasons. Firstly, they did not have enough blood samples and secondly the cost of transporting health care workers to a central site for training was prohibitive. Without appropriate training, health care workers may not have been using the Haemoglobin Colour Scale properly and each worker may have interpreted the results slightly differently. This would have meant that there would not have been high agreement between two workers on the same sample (inter-rater reliability). Also if each worker interpreted the result differently then the data would have lacked validity. For example if health care workers did not understand that they needed to always evaluate blood samples away from bright light, the results may have simply indicated the degree of sunshine in the place where the measurement was taken.

2 The authors developed an alternative training protocol that ensured that each health care worker used the Haemoglobin Colour Scale in the same way, but was also practical within the resource constraints. In particular the written instructions were complemented by a 'cartoon' version to aid comprehension and after a demonstration health care workers practised on a smaller number of blood samples. The effectiveness of the training was then tested by comparing the trainees' results with reference data of known haemoglobin. This ensures validity. Although not reported in the extract, the agreement between observers for the same blood sample could have been calculated. This would have provided an estimate of inter-rater reliability. The authors conclude that continued monitoring of health care workers on an individual basis is essential to ensure good measurement of haemoglobin in this context.

Types and sources of data

There are several different types of data that are relevant to the measurement of disease within a population. For the purposes of evaluation, they can be classified here as routine, *ad hoc* and standardized data.

Routine data

These data are collected systematically for a variety of purposes, often related to methods of paying health care providers. They may include hospital episode statistics or insurance claims databases. Routine data and the mechanisms by which they are collected were developed for particular purposes. This may restrict the choice of variables, the method of recording and the quality of the data themselves. Data used for billing can be cross-referenced with methods of identifying the patients and procedures concerned, along with other indicators of cost such as duration of stay and the cost of consumables. They do not necessarily include details of the severity of the patient's condition or co-morbidity.

Ad hoc data

These data are not usually collected systematically. They come from a variety of sources (such as general practice notes) and are recorded for many different purposes. Ad hoc data include information that is considered to be relevant to particular patients within the terms of particular consultations. Although some measurements are standardized (blood pressure, for instance), overall these data are limited by the very individual nature of the consultation. At the time they are collected, there is usually no plan to compare data from different patients' GP consultations and little effort is put into standardizing data collection or recording. Where ad hoc data are to be used for health care evaluation, it may be necessary to derive an index/scale or score composed of a number of variables.

Specially collected standardized data

When data are collected for special purposes, such as a trial or survey, much effort is put into the collection procedure. Trained observers, rigorously validated questionnaires and carefully standardized measuring procedures are used. These measurements should be comparable between different patients, different practitioners and different places.

There are a number of benefits and drawbacks of using data from these different sources. Activity 3.4 will give you the opportunity to think through some of these advantages and disadvantages.

Activity 3.4

List some advantages and disadvantages of using routine, *ad hoc* or specially collected standardized data to evaluate health care. Consider both the quantity and quality of data that might be available.

↻ **Feedback**

You may have considered the advantages and disadvantages shown in Table 3.2.

Table 3.2 Advantages and disadvantages of routine, ad hoc and standardized data

	Advantages	Disadvantages
Routine data	Lots of routine data exist; they have been collected in most developed health care systems, on a great many cases	Problems may arise when routine data are used to answer research questions beyond those for which they were collected
	As the data already exist there is no need to spend time collecting them; research questions can be answered more quickly	The quality of routine data often leaves much to be desired; if they have been collected for administrative or financial purposes, they may not be accurate enough for clinical case mix or outcome measurements
	If the evaluation seeks to measure a major, common outcome (e.g. mortality) and the disease is common, routine data may provide all the information that you need	They may be regarded as of minor importance by clinicians with the result that they may lack accuracy and completeness and be of low validity
		Severity and co-morbidity are very difficult to measure with confidence; for example, even such important co-morbidities as diabetes mellitus or renal failure are often omitted from routine records because only the principal diagnoses have been recorded
		Only a few outcomes can be recorded and coded routinely; these are, for example, in-hospital mortality and certain complications such as thromboses
		There is usually a lack of comparability between different institutions
Ad hoc data	They may be specific to the question being asked	Ad hoc data are often not collected centrally and it can be time consuming or expensive to obtain them
	It may be possible to contact original sources and improve completeness and quality	Depending on the nature of the data, they may represent fewer patients than routine data; however some common end-points, e.g. blood pressure, may be recorded for large numbers of patients
	Clinicians who collect this information may be personally interested in the outcomes that it measures; they would then have a personal interest in ensuring that it is accurate and complete	Several different scales or indices may be used to record ad hoc data. It can be difficult to relate such data, even where they relate to a similar condition, when they are collected from different sources

	The information already exists and this should speed up the process of evaluation	
Specially collected (standardized) data	Once the evaluation question has been stated clearly and the appropriate outcomes chosen, it becomes clear exactly which data are necessary	This information does not exist routinely and it can take a considerable period of time to collect and check it
	Quality control mechanisms can be incorporated into the design of the evaluation and improve accuracy and precision	This can be an expensive procedure
	The data will be appropriate to the analysis techniques as both have been chosen together	

Standardization of data

Standardization is a technique that can be used to adjust the measured outcomes to allow for different levels of a confounding variable such as age or sex (or both). If all other considerations are equal, you would expect the population with the higher proportion of elderly people to have the higher death rate. It is therefore necessary to adjust the outcomes to take account of this. Note that this is a different type of standardization to that referred to above (i.e. a standardized questionnaire meaning that everyone is asked the same questions in the same way).

Direct standardization applies the death rates occurring in the study population to the standard population. Indirect standardization performs the reverse process and applies the death rates occurring in the standard population to the study population.

National systems of registration

In many countries, information about certain diseases must be collected by law. This is a good example of routinely collected data. Most nations require that all deaths are registered, often with a medically certified cause of death. The accuracy of this information depends on the quality of the medical diagnosis and the completeness of registration. Mortality statistics in the UK are collected by the local registrars and forwarded to the Office of National Statistics. Skilled clerks then code the recorded causes of death using the ICD. This classification system is currently in its tenth revision. The data are published and presented in terms of mortality rates.

Quality of data

Whatever the source of the data, their quality and usefulness can vary considerably. This depends on a number of factors including:

- the accuracy of the measurement;
- completeness of registration;
- precision of coding;
- ability to retrieve data.

Summary

In this chapter you have considered the range of ways in which disease can be measured. These can be based on clinical criteria (such as ICD), direct measures (such as blood pressure) or self-, clinician- or proxy-reported questionnaire measures. All measures of disease should be reliable and valid and, for questionnaire measures, respondent burden and cross-cultural equivalence should also be considered. Measures of disease can be used as measures of outcome or as a way of controlling for confounding factors by assessing case-mix. Reliability and validity of disease measures can be threatened by a range of factors, including discrepancies between raters, use of inappropriate proxies and local misunderstandings of protocols. You have also considered the advantages and disadvantages of a variety of sources of data.

References

Bowling A (1997) *Measuring health: a review of quality of life measurement scales* (2nd edn). Buckingham: Open University Press.
Bowling A (2001) *Measuring disease* (2nd edn). Buckingham: Open University Press.
Calvo FA, Berrocal A, Pevez C, Romero F, Vega E, Cusi R, Visaga M, de la Cruz RA and Alarcon GS (1999) Self-administered joint counts in rheumatoid arthritis: comparison with standard joint counts. *The Journal of Rheumatology* 16: 536–9.
Charlson ME, Pompei P, Ales KL and McKenzie CR (1987) A new method of classifying prognostic comorbidity in longitudinal studies: development and validation. *Journal of Chronic Diseases* 40: 373–83.
Cohen J (1977) *Statistical power analysis for the behavioural sciences*. New York: Academic Press.
Criteria Committee of the New York Heart Association (1964) *Diseases of the heart and blood vessels: nomenclature and criteria for diagnosis* (6th edn). Boston, MA: Little, Brown.
Deyo RA, Diehr P and Patrick DL (1991) Reproducibility and responsiveness of health status measures: statistics and strategies for evaluation. *Controlled Clinical Trials* 12(Suppl. 4): 142–58.
Donaldson RJ and Donaldson LJ (1994) *Essential public health medicine*. Dordrecht: Kluwer.
Dujardin B, Clarysse G, Mentens H, De Schampheleire I and Kulker R (1993) How accurate is maternal height measurement in Africa? *International Journal of Gynaecology and Obstetrics* 41: 139–45.
Fitzpatrick R, Davey C, Buxton MJ and Jones DR (1998) Evaluating patient-based outcome measures for use in clinical trials. *Health Technology Assessment* 2: 14.
Gosling R, Walraven G, Fandinding M, Bailey R, Mitchell Lewis S *et al.* (2000) Training health workers to assess anaemia with the WHO haemoglobin colour scale. *Tropical Medicine and International Health* 5: 214–21.

Greenfield *et al.* (1993) The importance of co-existent disease in the occurrence of postoperative complications and one-year recovery in patients undergoing total hip replacement. Comorbidity and outcomes after hip replacement. *Medical Care* 31: 141–54.

Kazis L, Anderson JJ and Meenan RF (1990) Effect sizes for interpreting changes in health status. *Medical Care* 27(Suppl. 3): 178–89.

Liang MH, Fossel AH and Larson MG (1990) Comparisons of five health status instruments for orthopaedic evaluation. *Medical Care* 28(7): 632–42.

Lohr KN, Aaronson NK, Alonso J, Burnam MA, Patrick DL, Perrin EB and Roberts JS (1996) Evaluating quality-of-life and health status instruments: development of scientific review criteria. *Clinical Therapeutics* 18: 979–92.

McCaskie AW, Brown AR, Thompson JR and Gregg PJ (1996) Radiological evaluation of the interfaces after cemented total hip replacement. Interobserver and intraobserver agreement. *Journal of Bone Joint Surgery* 78-B: 191–4.

McDowell I and Jenkinson C (1996) Development standards for health measures. *Journal of Health Services Research and Policy* 1: 238–46.

Melzack R (1975) The McGill Pain Questionnaire: major properties and scoring methods. *Pain* 1: 277.

Melzack R (1987) The short-form McGill Questionnaire. *Pain* 30: 191–7.

Melzack R and Torgerson WS (1971) On the language of pain. *Anesthesiology* 34: 50.

Scientific Advisory Committee of the Medical Outcomes Trust (2002) Assessing health status and quality-of-life instruments: attributes and review criteria. *Quality of Life Research* 11: 193–205.

WHO (World Health Organization) (1980) *International classification of impairments, disabilities and handicaps*. Geneva: WHO.

WHO (World Health Organization) (2001) *International classification of functioning, disability and health*. Geneva: WHO.

4 Measuring health status and health-related quality of life

Overview

You now have an understanding of the techniques available for measuring disease and you have considered how these data might be obtained. In this chapter you will consider measures of health status and health-related quality of life (HRQL). You will learn about the conceptual basis of HRQL and how it differs from the types of measure we considered in the previous chapter, how generic measures differ from disease-specific measures and some of the ways in which HRQL measures are used. You will also discover some of the issues involved in cross-cultural application of measures of HRQL.

Learning objectives

After working through this chapter, you will be able to:

- describe the concept of HRQL
- explain the differences between generic and disease-specific measures and when each is appropriate for use
- critically appraise a range of measures of health status and HRQL and describe their appropriate use in health care evaluation
- outline the main issues in applying measures cross-culturally

Key terms

Disease-specific measures Instruments that focus on the particular aspects of the disease being studied.

Generic measures Instruments that measure general aspects of a person's health, such as mobility, sleeping and appetite.

Health-related quality of life The impact of the condition on the social functioning of a person, partly determined by the person's environment.

Index measures Measures of health that include a number of different health dimensions and aggregates them into a single score.

Profile measures Measures of health that include a number of health dimensions and produces a range of scores representing these different dimensions.

What is HRQL?

HRQL is generally considered to be subjective (i.e. it reflects the individuals' perception of their health and its impact) and multidimensional (i.e. it is based on a broad definition of health and includes more than simply physical health). One useful definition of HRQL is 'the impact of a perceived health state on an individual's potential to live a subjectively fulfilling life' (Bullinger *et al.* 1993). However, there is no universally accepted agreement over the domains that are included in conceptual models of HRQL. Most authors agree that it includes aspects of physical, psychological and social health and often these are described in terms of limitation in activities (e.g. Short-Form-36 (SF-36), WHO Quality of Life Group Scale (WHO-QOL), Nottingham Health Profile (NHP), Sickness Impact Profile (SIP)). Pain (e.g. SF-36, NHP), vitality or energy (SF-36, NHP), cognition and general health perceptions (SF-36, WHOQOL) are also sometimes included. HRQL is also sometimes described in terms of capacity or opportunity for health (Bergner 1985; Patrick and Bergner 1990; Patrick and Erickson 1993). However, this component is difficult to operationalize and is rarely included in instruments to measure HRQL.

Within the literature the terms HRQL, quality of life (QoL), health status and functional ability are often used interchangeably, although they actually describe different concepts. In general, health status describes the patient's health and may include signs, symptoms or functional disabilities caused by the disease. In contrast, HRQL refers to the impact of this state on the person's life. HRQL is generally considered to be more specific than QoL and refers to the impact of a health condition or intervention whereas QoL may also have a number of other influences, such as environmental or socioeconomic factors. Researchers will continue to debate the conceptual detail of these terms and related questions such as how HRQL differs from 'happiness' or 'well-being'. However, it is important that within health care evaluation investigators understand the broad distinctions and choose measures that are appropriate for the question under evaluation.

Activity 4.1 will give you an opportunity to consider why you might want to include a measure of HRQL in an evaluation of health care (in addition to measures of disease that we discussed in Chapter 3).

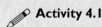 **Activity 4.1**

Imagine you are planning an evaluation of a treatment for diabetes. One outcome of interest might be blood glucose level (a measure of impairment), but you might also measure health status or HRQL. Why would HRQL be a useful outcome measure?

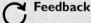 **Feedback**

There are several reasons why outcomes such as HRQL are important in health care evaluation. Blood glucose levels are an important clinical outcome, but do not tell you anything about the patient's functioning, well-being, or how they feel at home or at work. It is now widely recognized that it is important to understand health and health care in terms of the patient's own experience. Measures of HRQL enable the impact of the disease or intervention to be evaluated from the patient's perspective. For example, disease measures and HRQL measures may show different results. Patients with clinic-ally mild symptoms may experience their illness as more distressing or disturbing than the clinical assessment would suggest. In diabetes, a patient may suffer from impotence which may mean that sexual well-being and QoL is reduced. Diabetic retinopathy may mean that the patient is unable to drive which may affect their ability to carry out activities of daily living and hence satisfaction and QoL. The need for frequent injections may be considered a stigma by some patients and thus reduce QoL. It is important to be able to measure this experience of the patient. In addition, greater emphasis on cost-effectiveness has created a need for measures of quality as well as quantity. HRQL instruments help to provide this. The use of HRQL instruments in cost-effectiveness analysis will be discussed later in Chapter 11.

Generic versus disease-specific measures

Measures of HRQL can be either generic or disease-specific. Generic measures are intended to be used with any condition and they include questions that are rele-vant to any type disease. Well-known generic measures of HRQL and health status include the SF-36 (Ware *et al.* 1993, 1994), NHP (Hunt 1984; Hunt *et al.* 1986) and WHOQOL (WHOQOL Group 1998). In contrast, disease-specific measures are designed to be used only with one condition and the questions are very specific to patients' experience with that particular disease. For example, the Stroke-Specific Quality of Life scale (SSQOL) is designed specifically to evaluate HRQL after a stroke (Williams *et al.* 1999). Some measures can also be described as 'site specific'. These instruments are designed to be applicable to a general area of disease, such as vision, but may not be specific to a particular disease. This type of questionnaire would therefore be appropriate for use with people with a visual impairment result-ing from a variety of diseases (e.g. cataract, macular degeneration, glaucoma etc). For example, the India Visual function Questionnaire (IND-VFQ) was developed to measure vision-related quality of life in India (Gupta *et al.* in press).

Generic and disease-specific measures both have advantages and disadvantages. Generic measures have broad coverage of conceptual domains. As a result they can be used with a variety of diseases and enable direct comparison across conditions. However, generic measures may not address specific content areas that are con-sidered to be particularly relevant for some conditions. Generic measures may not be as sensitive to the change in HRQL resulting from the treatment (responsive-ness). Disease-specific measures have content that is more focused and therefore tend to have greater sensitivity to change. However, because the measures are only applicable to a particular condition it is not possible to compare a variety of conditions using the same measure.

The choice between generic and disease-specific measures depends on the nature of the evaluation. A full evaluation would include both, but this may require more questionnaires to be completed and there may therefore be more burden placed on the patient. In some evaluations, the intervention would not be expected to show very large effects on HRQL (e.g. if the condition was relatively mild). In these situations a generic measure may not be sensitive enough to show the effects and a disease-specific measure would be preferable. In other situations, where it is necessary to compare the evaluation of a range of conditions (e.g. for decisions about resource allocation), a generic measure might be preferable, so that each condition can be evaluated on the same scale.

 Activity 4.2

Read the following extract from an article by two well known HRQL researchers (Patrick and Deyo 1989). The extract refers to two acronyms which are not fully explained in the text. The HAQ refers to the Health Assessment Questionnaire and the QWB refers to the Quality of Well-Being Scale. Consider the following questions:

1   How could you combine generic and disease-specific outcome measures within a particular study?
2   How could you modify an existing generic instrument so that it is more relevant to the population under investigation?
3   What other ways could you include a wide range of HRQL domains as outcomes?

Models for using generic and disease-specific measures

Four different models seem relevant in examining the use of generic and disease-specific measures to date. Examples of each approach are described below.

Separate generic and disease-specific measures

The first approach is to include both generic and disease-specific measures in the same investigation even though the concepts covered by the different instruments may overlap substantially. An example of this approach is the 6-month, randomized, double-blind study of auranofin therapy for the treatment of patients with rheumatoid arthritis (Bombardier *et al.* 1986). The arthritis-specific measure used in the trial was the HAQ, which specifies eight areas of daily function (e.g., hygiene) each with two to three activities (e.g., take a tub bath). Patients report difficulty in performing each activity during the past week with scores from 3 ('unable to do') to 0 ('without any difficulty') and lower (better) values are raised if aids, devices, or help from another are needed.

This trial also incorporated the generic QWB, which classifies patients into one of four or five given categories of performance (e.g., 'had help with self-care activities') and the least desirable symptom or problem for each day. Both functional status categories and symptoms are assigned a value using psychometric scaling techniques that have been elicited from both general populations and arthritis patients yielding an overall QWB score for each patient on a scale from 0 (death) to 1.0 (maximum health).

The HAQ and the QWB showed comparable sensitivity to treatment, although the instruments have different content, length, mode of administration, and method of scoring. Previous clinical findings of the efficacy of auranofin were corroborated in the trial, and both the HAQ and the QWB measures were consistent with more traditional clinical measures, such as the number of tender joints, grip strength, and erythrocyte sedimentation rate.

Interpretation of the benefit associated with auranofin proved similarly difficult with the HAQ or QWB (Thompson *et al.* 1988). On the HAQ, patients receiving auranofin reduced their disability by an average of 0.31 points. The authors concluded that 0.17 points of the 0.31-point improvement would have been achieved by placebo alone, and the net effect was equivalent to all auranofin patients improving from being able to walk outdoors on level ground 'with much difficulty' to 'with some difficulty.' Similarly, the 0.020 overall gain on the QWB was judged equivalent to all auranofin patients improving on the physical activity scale from 'moving one's own wheelchair without help' to 'walking with physical limitations,' again of 0.017 points. In contrast to the HAQ, the QWB did not detect any placebo effects, possibly because of the generic nature of the instrument.

The authors of this study concluded that the advantages of using the HAQ were ease of administration, extensive validation, and proven sensitivity to therapeutic efficacy. The QWB required more care in administration and as not explicitly concerned with rheumatoid arthritis patients. The value weights assigned to the QWB, however, permitted the authors to examine adverse clinical effects, of therapy that could be compared directly. Clearly, a trade-off is involved between the detection and weighting of different intervention effects when using generic and specific measures.

Generic versus modified generic measures

The second approach to examining the relative strengths of generic and disease specific measures is to compare a generic instrument and a generic instrument modified for the specific population of interest. This approach has been used in the study of head injury and in the assessment of back pain. Both investigations modified the SIP to improve its sensitivity to the clinical condition being evaluated. The study of head injury (Temkin *et al.* 1989) added items to the SIP to capture head injury sequelae and behaviors typical of young adults who experience head injury most frequently. These items were reweighted to be included in the global measures derived from the SIP.

In the study of back pain, the authors selected 24 of 136 items that they felt were most appropriate for back pain from eight of 12 different SIP categories. Each item was scored as a (0, 1) variable. The phrase 'because of my back' was added to each statement to distinguish dysfunction attributed to back pain from that due to other causes. Scores on this scale ranged from 0 to 24 with higher scores representing worse dysfunction. Global SIP scores, on the other hand, include a 45-item physical dimension, 49-item psychosocial dimension, and 53 items in independent categories of eating, work, sleep and rest, household management, and recreation and pastimes.

A separate study (Deyo and Centor 1986) compared the complete SIP with the version modified for back pain (Roland Scale) in a clinical trial with 203 subjects, most of whom (79%) had acute back pain. Both the overall SIP and the Roland scale showed significant correlations between change scores and changes in self-rated improvement, clinician-rated improvement, spine flexion, and resumption of full activities. The Roland Scale showed slightly better discrimination between improvers and non-improvers than either the overall SIP or its physical dimension score. The 'pruned' condition-specific Roland Scale was at least as responsive as the lengthier SIP in both discrimination and in the quantification of changes. Furthermore, reliability and construct validity of the shorter scale were comparable to those of the complete SIP.

Generic with disease-specific supplement

The third approach is to use a generic health status instrument with a condition-specific supplement. This is similar to the first approach except that the condition-specific measure is constructed to have a different conceptual basis and minimal overlap with the generic measure. The intention is not to measure the same concepts as a generic measure with specific reference to a medical condition, but to capture the additional, specific concerns of patients with the condition that are not contained in generic measures.

This approach has been used in the study of patients with inflammatory bowel disease (IBD). In a study of 150 patients with Crohn's disease and ulcerative colitis, the SIP was administered to measure functional status. A 21-item Rating Form of IBD Patient Concerns (RFIPC) was constructed by eliciting items through semistructured interviews concerning the worries, fears, or concerns that IBD patients might have. Although these concerns were IBD-specific, four items—bowel control, pain, sexual performance, and feelings of aloneness—are also measured in terms of behavioral dysfunction in the SIP. Items on the RFIPC were rated by patients from 0 to 100 (0 = not at all concerned to 100 = a great deal concerned) on a visual analogue scale, and an average score of all concerns (sumscore) was calculated.

In cross-sectional comparisons, both the SIP and RFIPC proved to be discriminating measures of health-related quality of life in patients with inflammatory bowel disease. The SIP was sensitive to different disease populations; patients with Crohn's reported more dysfunction (overall SIP = 8.6) than patients with ulcerative colitis (overall SIP = 5.2). The RFIPC showed a similar pattern of concerns between the two patient groups, although inpatients compared with outpatients reported considerably higher concerns with dying, intimacy, body image, being a burden, and finances. This pattern of concerns is consistent with the greater severity of disease activity among inpatients. The correlation between the overall RFIPC score and the overall SIP score was 0.46 (P = .0002), a moderate correlation indicating a strong, but not predictive, relationship between behavioral dysfunction and worries and concerns in this patient population. Incorporating the SIP in this study permitted comparisons with other healthy and condition-specific population . . . showing that IBD patients report moderate overall dysfunction comparable to adult patients with rheumatoid arthritis (unstandardized for age and sex). IBD patients however, appear to report somewhat higher (worse) psychosocial dimension scores.

Batteries of specific measures

The battery approach refers to collections of specific measures that are scored independently and reported as individual scores. Although generic instruments may be included in health status batteries, collections of specific measures are more often used. Batteries are common in clinical trials and epidemiologic investigations, where entire scales, subscales, or individual items from the best available instruments are administered and effects are tested for each measure in the battery.

One example of this approach is a double-blind, randomized trial of three antihypertensive agents in primary hypertension (Croog et al. 1986). Separate measures were included of well-being, physical symptoms, sexual function, work performance, emotional status, cognitive function, social participation, and life satisfaction. Patients taking captopril, one of the three drugs in the trial, scored better on measures of general well-being work performance, and life satisfaction. Fortunately for the investigators, measures included in the battery did not yield conflicting results, e.g., positive for sexual function and negative for work performance. The battery approach, as illustrated by this trial, does not yield an overall score for summarizing net effects nor provide any indication of the relative importance of each dimension of health that would permit inter-measure comparisons.

Feedback

1 Generic and disease-specific measures are often used in the same investigation. The disease-specific measure may be shorter and easier to administer and it may have extensive evidence of reliability and validity in the particular condition that is being evaluated. The generic measure may allow direct comparisons to be made between treatments or between conditions. Before you use any measure in an evaluation you must be sure that it has acceptable psychometric properties (i.e. reliability, validity and responsiveness).

2 You could modify an existing generic instrument so that it is more sensitive to the condition being evaluated. This could involve modifying items (i.e. questions), adding new items or selecting a subset of thee existing items. Note however that the scores derived from the modified generic scale cannot be compared with scores obtained from the original generic scale. Although the extract does not make this explicit, you would need to ensure that any modified version of the questionnaire was rigorously tested for reliability, validity and responsiveness before using it. Often authors who have modified a generic scale fail to retest its psychometric properties.

3 An alternative approach would be to incorporate a battery of measures into your investigation. For example, you could include separate measures for each domain (e.g. physical symptoms, social function, life satisfaction etc.). This approach would mean that you had a separate score for each instrument in the battery, but interpretation of these different scores can be complex, as you would not know the relative importance of each instrument.

Types of HRQL measure

Most measures of HRQL are standardized instruments. This means that they consist of a predetermined set of items, all the respondents answer the same items and rate them using the same response scale. The format and order of items is also usually predetermined. Standardized measures can produce a single overall score (a health index) or a series of separate scores, one for each domain (a health profile). Some index measures also include preference weightings known as 'utilities' for each item. The SF-36 (Ware *et al.* 1993, 1994) is a well-known example of a profile measure. It consists of 36 items, each rated on a Likert-type scale. The items represent eight conceptual domains: physical functioning, role limitations due to physical problems, role limitations due to emotional problems, social functioning, mental health, energy, pain and general health perceptions. These are combined into two summary scores: physical health and mental health. The Euroqol (EQ-5D) instrument (Euroqol Group 1990) is an example of an index measure. It consists of five questions representing mobility, self-care, usual activity, pain and mood. Each question is rated on a three-point response scale (Level 1 'no problems'; Level 2 'some problems'; Level 3 'inability or extreme problems'). This generates 245 health states, including death and unconsciousness, for example the health state 11111 would represent no problem on any of the domains or perfect health. Weighted preference values have been obtained from national and international samples and these are applied to the health states to generate an index score. An alternative approach to measuring HRQL is to use individualized instruments where respondents choose the domains that are important to them, rather than rate a standard set of items. However, this type of measure is rarely used in evaluation of health care because it is not possible to compare scores for different patients.

There are advantages and disadvantages to both health indices and health profiles. Health indices generate a single score and allow a straightforward comparison between the measurements from two or more different health care interventions. In contrast, the dimension scores from health profiles reflect the multidimensional nature of HRQL and produce a more comprehensive picture of health. However, comparisons between two or more conditions or interventions can be complex, particularly when some domains show effect and others do not.

Some measures of HRQL are also used to combine assessment of QoL with an indicator of the *quantity* of life. These are called *utility measures*. The questionnaire items are used to form a set of health states, a 'utility' value is derived and this is applied to the health states produced from the survey. Utilities are population-based preferences for various health states. Utility measures are often used in evaluating cost-effectiveness through, for example, the use of quality-adjusted life years (QALYs). The various methods by which utilities can be obtained are discussed in Chapter 12.

Cross-cultural issues

It is essential that all measures of HRQL are appropriate for each context in which they are used. Where international comparisons are made within an evaluation of an intervention or where a measure is used in a culture that is different to the one for which it was originally developed, cross-cultural equivalence needs to be demonstrated. This is a complex and time-consuming process that involves testing the equivalence of the language, conceptual content and response scales and also re-evaluating psychometric properties.

Bullinger *et al.* (1996) provide a useful summary of three main ways that cross-cultural instruments can be developed. Firstly in the sequential approach the instrument is initially developed and validated in the original language. It is then translated and back-translated and the resulting versions are rated for conceptual equivalence, colloquial language and clarity. The new instrument is then tested for feasibility, acceptability and comprehension. The equivalence of the response scales is then tested statistically and the psychometric properties of the instrument are then re-evaluated. The International Quality of Life (IQOLA) project (Ware *et al.* 1995) used this approach to develop cross-cultural applications for the SF-36. Secondly, cross-cultural instruments can be developed in parallel with the original instrument. In this approach, the international relevance of items is determined at the beginning of the development process and the final set of items are chosen because they are applicable across a variety of national contexts. The single set of items are then translated and back-translated and the psychometric properties of each language version evaluated. The European Organization for Research on Treatment of Cancer (EORTC) quality of life group used this approach to develop the EORTC quality of life questionnaire (EORTC 1983; van Dam *et al.* 1984;

Aaronson 1986, 1987, 1993; Aaronson *et al.* 1988, 1991, 1993). This instrument consists of a core set of items with additional disease-specific modules that can be used in conjunction with the core instrument. Finally, cross-cultural instruments can be developed simultaneously. This approach adopts a common core of items that are applicable across cultures but then acknowledges that there are additional country-specific items. After translation and back-translation, each country-specific version is evaluated for its psychometric properties. The WHOQOL Group (1998) used this approach to develop the WHOQOL questionnaire. In order to compare the psychometric properties in each country or culture it is essential that the studies are comparable in terms of the patient groups and study designs (Bullinger *et al.* 1996).

Summary

In this chapter you have examined the need for measures of health status and HRQL and seen that these are an important complement to the disease measures discussed in Chapter 3. Generic measures allow comparisons between different conditions but may lack sensitivity, whereas disease-specific measures may be more sensitive but can only be used with a particular condition. Generic and disease-specific measures can be used together. If a measure is adapted or modified (either to make a generic measure more applicable to a particular condition or to adapt an instrument for use in another culture) the instrument's psychometric properties (reliability, validity and responsiveness) must be re-evaluated before it is used in the evaluation of health care.

References

Aaronson NK (1986) Methodological issues in psychosocial oncology with special reference to clinical trials, in Ventafridda V *et al.* (eds) *Assessment of quality of life and cancer treatment.* Amsterdam: Elsevier.

Aaronson NK (1987) *EORTC Protocol 15861: development of a core quality-of-life questionnaire for use in cancer clinical trials.* Brussels: EORTC Data Centre.

Aaronson NK (1993) The EORTC QLQ-c30: a quality of life instrument for use in international clinical trials in oncology. *Quality of Life Research* 2: 51.

Aaronson NK, Bullinger M and Ahmedzai S (1988) A modular approach to quality of life assessment in cancer clinical trials. *Recent Results in Cancer Research* 111: 231–49.

Aaronson NK, Ahmedzai S and Bullinger M *et al.* (1991) The EORTC core quality of life questionnaire: interim results of an international field study, in Osoba D (ed.) *Effect of cancer on quality of life.* Boca Raton, CA: CRC Press.

Aaronson NK, Ahmedzai S, Bergman B *et al.* (1993) The European Organization for Research and Treatment of Cancer QLQ-C30: a quality of life instrument for use in international trials in oncology. *Journal of the National Cancer Institute* 85: 365–76.

Bergner M. (1985) Measurement of health status. *Medical Care* 23: 696–704.

Bombardier C, Ware J and Rausell IJ *et al.* (1986) Auranofin therapy and quality of life in patients with rheumatoid arthritis: results of a multicenter trial. *American Journal of Medicine* 81: 565.

Bullinger M, Anderson R, Cella D and Aaronson N (1993) Developing and evaluating cross-cultural instruments from minimum requirements to optimal models. *Quality of Life Research* 2: 451–9.

Bullinger M, Power MJ, Aaronson NK, Cella DF and Anderson RT (1996) Creating and evaluating cross-cultural instruments, in Spilker B (ed.) *Quality of life and pharmaco-economics in clinical trials*. Philadelphia, PA: Lippincott-Raven Publishers.

Croog SH, Levine S, Testa MA *et al.* (1986) The effects of antihypertensive therapy on the quality of life. *New England Journal of Medicine* 314: 1657.

Deyo RA and Centor RM (1986) Assessing the responsiveness of functional scales to clinical change: an analogy to diagnostic test performance. *Journal of Chronic Diseases* 11: 897.

EORTC (European Organization for Research on Treatment of Cancer) (1983) *Quality of life: methods of measurement and related areas*. Proceedings of the 4th Workshop EORTC Study Group. Odense, Denmark: Odense University Hospital.

Euroqol Group (1990) Euroqol: a new facility for the measurement of health related quality of life. *Health Policy* 16: 199–208.

Gupta SK, Viswaneth MD, Thulasiraj MBA, Murthy MD, Lamping DL, Smith SC, Donoghue M and Fletcher AE (in press) Psychometric evaluation of the Indian Vision Function Questionnaire. *British Journal of Opthalmology*.

Hunt SM (1984) Nottingham health profile, in Wenger NK *et al.* (eds) *Assessment of quality of life in clinical trials of cardiovascular therapies*. New York: Le Jacq.

Hunt SM, McEwan J and McKenna SO (1986) *Measuring health status*. Beckenham: Croom Helm.

Patrick DL and Bergner M. (1990) Measurement of health status in the 1990s. *Annual Review of Public Health* 11: 165–83.

Patrick DL and Deyo RA (1989) Generic and disease-specific measures in assessing health status and quality of life. *Medical Care* 27: S217–232.

Patrick DL and Erickson P (1993) *Quality of life, assessment of health and allocation of resources*. Oxford: Oxford University Press.

Temkin NMA Jr, Dikmen S *et al.* (1989) Development and evaluation of modifications to the Sickness Impact Profile for head injury. *Journal of Clinical Epidemiology* 41: 47.

Thompson MS, Read LJ, Hutchings HC *et al.* (1988) The cost effectiveness of auranofin: results of a randomised clinical trial. *Journal of Rheumatology* 16: 35.

van Dam FSAM, Linssen CAG and Couzijin AL (1984) Evaluating quality of life in cancer clinical trials, in Buyse ME *et al.* (eds) *Cancer clinical trials: methods and practice*. New York: Oxford University Press.

Ware JE, Snow KK, Kosinski M and Gandek B (1993) *SF-36 manual and interpretation guide*. Boston, MA: The Health Institute, New England Medical Center.

Ware JE, Kosinski MA and Keller SD (1994) *SF-36 physical and mental component summary measures: a user's manual*. Boston, MA: The Health Institute, New England Medial Center.

Ware JE Jr, Keller SD, Gandek B, Brazier JE and Sullivan M (1995) Evaluating translations of health status questionnaires: methods from the IQOLA Project. *International Journal of Technology Assessment in Health Care* 11: 525–51.

Williams LS, Weinberger M, Harris LE, Clark DO and Biller H (1999) Development of a stroke-specific quality of life scale. *Stroke* 30: 1362–9.

WHOQOL Group (1998) The World Health Organization Quality of Life Assessment (WHOQOL): development and general psychometric properties. *Social Science and Medicine* 46(12): 1569–85.

SECTION 3

Evaluating effectiveness

5

Association and causality

Overview

Now that you have considered how to measure various aspects of health, this and the next four chapters will explore how to determine the effectiveness of health care interventions. This chapter will introduce the concepts of statistical association and causality and will discuss some of the factors that can interfere with this relationship.

Learning objectives

By the end of this chapter you will be able to:

- **explain what is meant by statistical association**
- **identify potential problems due to bias and confounding**
- **discuss the need to consider validity and generalizability in study design**
- **critically appraise evidence suggesting a causal relationship between intervention and outcome**

Key terms

Causality The relating of causes to the effects they produce.

Confounding Situation in which an estimate of the association between a risk factor (exposure) and outcome is distorted because of the association of the exposure with another risk factor (a confounding variable) for the outcome under study.

External validity (generalizability) The extent to which the results of a study can be generalized to the population from which the sample was drawn.

Internal validity The extent to which the results of a study are not affected by bias and confounding.

Statistical association The demonstration that the outcome varies with the intervention that is being evaluated.

Statistical significance The likelihood that an association can be explained by chance alone.

Effectiveness and efficacy

Effectiveness describes the benefits of interventions measured by improvements in health outcomes in a typical population (e.g. in a general hospital or treatment centre setting). Most health care evaluation is conducted in these settings, though differences in populations may still mean that results from the use of an intervention in one place may not apply somewhere else.

In contrast, *efficacy* describes how much health improvement can be obtained from an intervention under ideal conditions (e.g. a specialist setting, such as a teaching hospital). These settings may be very different from the circumstances of the majority of patients with the same disease. For example, patients included may be either more or less ill than the majority of patients. The health care staff may not behave in the same way as staff caring for patients who are not in the study. For example, they may be more alert to particular adverse events of therapy or may take a greater interest in patient follow-up.

Demonstrating a statistical association

Statistical association is the demonstration that the outcome varies with the intervention that is being evaluated (i.e. that the outcome is either better or worse in the treated group than in the non-treated group). Demonstrating a statistical association is a central part of health care evaluation. However, establishing that there is a statistical association between the intervention and the outcome does not mean that there is a causal relationship between the two. To show that a valid statistical association exists, it is necessary to demonstrate that:

- the outcome is related to the intervention (i.e. the outcome is *associated* with the intervention);
- the association is not simply due to chance;
- the association is not due to bias or confounding.

The association between two variables (e.g. an intervention and an outcome) can be measured using a variety of epidemiological and statistical tests. The choice of test depends on a number of factors that are specific to individual studies and the type of data collected. Often-used epidemiological measures include odds ratios and risk ratios. Examples of statistical tests that might be used to measure association include t-test, analysis of variance (ANOVA) and correlations for continuous data or a chi square test for categorical data.

The likelihood that any association is due simply to chance is evaluated using a statistical test of significance. This is based on probability theory and usually tests the null hypothesis that there is no difference between the two groups other than the difference that would be seen by chance alone. The p-value represents the probability that the difference between two groups is due to chance. By convention $p < 0.05$ is usually taken to mean that the difference is greater than would be expected simply by chance (though sometimes more stringent criteria are used, for example $p < 0.01$ or $p < 0.001$). This is described as the difference being 'statistically significant'. A p-value of 0.05 means that 5 times in 100 the difference would be expected to occur by chance. A statistically significant result means that it is unlikely that the findings were due purely to chance. However, it does not entirely exclude the possibility that the result may occur by chance. Therefore although a *p*-value may be very small it is not usually zero.

An alternative way of considering whether a result is likely to be due to chance is by considering the confidence intervals around the value. A confidence interval is the range within which the true value is likely to occur. Usually investigators report the 95 per cent confidence interval, which means that 95 times out of 100 the true value will lie between the upper and lower value of the confidence interval.

The concept of statistical significance is linked to sample size and the concept of statistical power. Statistical power can be described as the degree of confidence that is required to obtain a statistically significant difference, if such a difference actually exists. This is usually set at 80, 90 or 95 per cent. By considering the size of the treatment effect that is expected, the required level of power and the acceptable level of statistical significance, the appropriate sample size can be calculated using statistical tables or various software packages.

This relationship between statistical significance, power and sample size means that a sample size that it is too small may mean that you have inadequate power to show a significant result, even if the effect is large. Conversely in very large samples a small effect may still be statistically significant. The magnitude of an effect is often measured using an 'effect size'. This is usually calculated using the formula $(\text{mean}_{\text{pre-treatment}} - \text{mean}_{\text{post-treatment}})/(\text{sd}_{\text{pre-treatment}})$.

A statistically significant finding does not tell us anything about the direction of the association (i.e. whether the intervention causes the outcome), nor does it give any indication of the influence of bias and confounding factors. Both of these will be considered later in this chapter.

Activity 5.1

1   What is a statistical association?
2   How would you decide if the association was due to chance alone?

Feedback

1   A statistical association exists when the outcome of a study is shown to vary with the intervention that is being investigated. That is, the outcome in one group is either better or worse than the other group. In order to show that an association is valid, the investigator must show that the likelihood that it is due to chance, bias or confounding has been minimized.

2   The likelihood that an apparent association is measured by chance may be measured by a statistical test of significance. The *p*-value represents the probability that the measured association is due to chance alone. If a finding is statistically significant, this means that it is unlikely that the finding is simply the result of chance, but it does not rule out the possibility that it is due to chance.

Internal validity

The extent to which a finding is free from bias and confounding factors is known as internal validity. Even if a finding is statistically significant it is still necessary to establish that the results are not caused by bias or confounding factors. Bias (or 'systematic error' as it is sometimes called) arises when groups of patients are different in ways that are not due simply to chance. It interferes with the degree of association that exists between a health care intervention and the outcome that is being tested and can cause either over- or underestimates of the degree of association. The following extract from Grimes and Schulz (2002) will help to explain some of the problems associated with different forms of bias.

 Selection bias

Are the groups similar in all important respects?

Selection bias stems from an absence of comparability between groups being studied. For example, in a cohort study, the exposed and unexposed groups differ in some important respect aside from the exposure. Membership bias is a type of selection bias: people who choose to be members of a group – e.g. joggers – might differ in important respects from others. For instance, both cohort and case-control studies initially suggested that jogging after myocardial infarction prevented repeat infarction. However, a randomised controlled trial failed to confirm this benefit (Sackett 1979). Those who chose to exercise might have differed in other important ways from those who did not exercise, such as diet, smoking, and presence of angina.

In case-control studies, selection bias implies that cases and controls differ importantly aside from the disease in question. Two types of selection bias have earned eponyms: Berkson and Neyman bias. Also known as an admission-rate bias, Berkson bias (or paradox) results from differential rates of hospital admission for cases and controls. Berkson initially thought that this phenomenon was due to presence of a simultaneous disease. Alternatively, knowledge of the exposure of interest might lead to an increased rate of admission to hospital . . .

Neyman bias is an incidence-prevalence bias. It arises when a gap in time occurs between exposure and selection of study participants. This bias crops up in studies of diseases that are quickly fatal, transient, or subclinical. Neyman bias creates a case group not representative of cases in the community. For example, a hospital-based case-control study of myocardial infarction and snow shovelling (the exposure of interest) would miss individuals who died in their driveways and thus never reached a hospital; this eventuality might greatly lower the odds ratio of infarction associated with this strenuous activity.

Other types of selection bias include unmasking (detection signal) and non-respondent bias. An exposure might lead to a search for an outcome, as well as the outcome itself. For example, oestrogen replacement therapy might cause symptomless endometrial cancer patients to bleed, resulting in initiation of diagnostic tests (Feinstein and Horowitz 1977). In this instance, the exposure unmasked the subclinical cancer, leading to a spurious increase in the odds ratio. In observational studies, non-respondents are different from respondents. Cigarette smokers are a case in point: smokers are less likely to return questionnaires than are non-smokers or pipe and cigar smokers.

Information bias

Has information been gathered in the same way?

Information bias, also known as observation, classification, or measurement bias, results from incorrect determination of exposure or outcome, or both. In a cohort study or randomised controlled trial, information about outcomes should be obtained the same way for those exposed and unexposed. In a case-control study, information about exposure should be gathered in the same way for cases and controls.

Information bias can arise in many ways. Some use the term ascertainment to describe gathering information in different ways. For example, an investigator might gather information about an exposure at bedside for a case but by telephone from a community control. Diagnostic suspicion bias implies that knowledge of a putative cause of disease might launch a more intensive search for the disease among those exposed, for example, preferentially searching for infection by HIV-I in intravenous drug users. Conversely, the presence of a disease might prompt a search for the putative exposure of interest. Another type of bias is family history bias, in which medical information flows differently to affected and unaffected family members. To minimise information bias, detail about exposures in case-control studies should be gathered by people who are unaware of whether the respondent is a case or a control. Similarly, in a cohort study with subjective outcomes, the observer should be unaware of the exposure status of each participant.

In case-control studies that rely on memory of remote exposures, recall bias is pervasive. Cases tend to search their memories to identify what might have caused their disease; healthy controls have no such motivation. Thus, better recall among cases is common.

Selection bias can be reduced by allocating patients to different treatment groups at random. If it is not possible to randomly allocate patients, then ensuring that each group is similar in terms of case-mix characteristics such as age, sex and severity of illness can help to prevent selection bias. It is always wise to measure the distribution of these case-mix variables in each group, even if patients were randomly allocated. It is then possible to demonstrate that the groups were equivalent in terms of patient characteristics.

Information bias can be reduced by ensuring that each group has the same information, the same follow-up and ideally the same tests. 'Blinding' of the interviewer (or investigator) prevents bias arising because the interviewer asked different questions of the different groups. For some treatments it may not be possible to achieve this (e.g. a patient's scar may make it obvious that they have had surgery). 'Blinding' the patient so that he or she does not know whether they received the new treatment or the standard treatment helps to reduce the bias related to the respondent (also known as placebo bias). By using placebos (i.e. an inert treatment that does not have a biological effect) it may be possible to 'blind' the patient to a particular drug treatment as the patient does not know if they've been given the active drug or the placebo. However, it may not be possible to 'blind' the patient for surgical treatments or for some social interventions.

Confounding is the result of differences in population structure and occurs when the result is due to a factor that is associated with both the intervention and is a risk factor for the outcome in its own right. Confounding variables can give the appearance of an association that does not exist or can prevent the study from identifying an association that really does exist (Hennekens and Buring 1987). Grimes and

Schulz (2002) describe confounding as being when 'A researcher attempts to relate an exposure to an outcome, but actually measures the effect of a third factor, termed a confounding variable'. The following extract by the same authors will help to explain some of the ways in which confounding can be controlled.

 ### Control for confounding

When selection bias or information bias exist in a study, irreparable damage results. Internal validity is doomed. By contrast, when confounding is present, this bias can be corrected, provided that confounding was anticipated and the requisite information gathered. Confounding can be controlled for before or after a study is done. The purpose of these approaches is to achieve homogeneity between study groups.

Restriction

The simplest approach is restriction (also called exclusion or specification). For example, if cigarette smoking is suspected to be a confounding factor, a study can enrol only non-smokers. Although this tactic avoids confounding, it also hinders recruitment (and thus power) and precludes extrapolation to smokers. Restriction might increase the internal validity of a study at the cost of poorer external validity.

Matching

Another way to control for confounding is pairwise matching. In a case-control study in which smoking is deemed a confounding factor, cases and controls can be matched by smoking status. For each case who smokes, a control who smokes is found. This approach, although often used by investigators, has two drawbacks. If matching is done on several potential confounding factors, the recruitment process can be cumbersome, and, by definition, one cannot examine the effect of a matched variable!

Stratification

Investigators can also control for confounding after a study has been completed. One approach is stratification. Stratification can be considered a form of post hoc restriction, done during the analysis rather than during the accrual phase of a study. For example, results can be stratified by levels of the confounding factor . . . The Mantel-Haenszel procedure (Mantel and Haenszel 1959) combines the various strata into a summary statistic that describes the effect . . .

Multivariate techniques

In multivariate techniques, mathematical modelling examines the potential effect of one variable while simultaneously controlling for the effect of many other factors. A major advantage of these approaches is that they can control for more factors that can stratification. For example, an investigator might use multivariate [techniques] to study the effect of oral contraceptives on ovarian cancer risk. In this way, they could simultaneously control for age, race, family history, parity, &c.

 ### Activity 5.2

Imagine that you are a researcher planning a study to compare a group of patients with arthritis of the hand who receive surgical arthroplasty with another group who receive steroid injections. On a separate piece of paper, complete Table 5.1 with definitions and examples of different kinds of bias. A worked example is given to start you off.

Table 5.1 Sources of bias in comparison of treatments for arthritis of the hand

Type of bias	Definition	Example
Selection bias	The two groups differ in some respect that is not the intervention under investigation	Might occur if patients who were more functionally limited were *selected* to receive the arthroplasty on the grounds that they were unlikely to benefit from the steroid injections
Information bias		
Confounding		

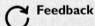 **Feedback**

Your completed version of Table 5.1 might resemble Table 5.2.

Table 5.2 Sources of bias in comparison of treatments for arthritis of the hand – solutions

Type of bias	Definition	Example
Selection bias	The two groups differ in some respect that is not the intervention under investigation	Examples might include: • Might occur if patients who were more functionally limited were *selected* to receive the arthroplasty on the grounds that they were unlikely to benefit from the steroid injections • If patients drop out of the study before it is complete or if they change treatments. If this happens more in one group than the other, this may result in selection bias as the two groups would be systematically different
Information bias	When the outcome is measured incorrectly or inaccurately or when the outcome is measured differently in the two groups. Also known as observation bias or measurement bias	Examples might include: • If patients in the arthroplasty group were reviewed more frequently in the clinic than patients in the injection group • If an interviewer treats patients from different study groups in a different manner. This might arise if the interviewer knew for example that the arthroplasty

Type of bias	Definition	Example
Information bias cont		was likely to cause limitations in use of the hand and also knew which treatment patients had received (because of the scarring from the surgery). Consequently, those patients who had received arthroplasty might be asked more searching questions related to functional ability • When participants report certain information because they know the treatment group to which they were allocated and also know the expected effects of the treatment. Patients will know whether they received surgery or injections and if they also know that arthroplasty of the hand may lead to more negative body image, they may be more likely to report the expected side-effect
Confounding	Occurs when the finding is the result of a third variable that is related to both the intervention and the outcome, but is not part of the way the intervention causes the outcome	Examples might include: • If the study demonstrates that people receiving arthroplasty had less functional ability in their hands, this may be due to the surgery but may also be due to other factors such as age. These additional factors would be confounding factors

Implications for planning a study

It is important to anticipate and try to avoid both bias and confounding. There are specific techniques that can be used to minimize these. Selection and information bias must be addressed before the data are collected whereas confounding can be addressed either before or after the data are collected (provided that the relevant data have been collected).

External validity

External validity is the extent to which the results can be applied to the wider population. A particular study can only measure the association between an intervention and outcomes in those patients that take part. To be of relevance to the wider population it is necessary to demonstrate that the results are generalizable. In general, external validity (or generalizability) is increased when the sample is representative of the wider population. However, it is important to show that a study has internal validity before attempting to show generalizability.

Demonstrating causality

Once a statistical association has been established, it is necessary to decide whether a causal relationship exists. The following extract by Grimes and Schulz (2002) will explain how to demonstrate a cause-effect relationship between an intervention and an outcome.

Judgment of associations: bogus, indirect, or real?

When statistical associations emerge from clinical research, the next step is to judge what type of association exists. Statistical associations do not necessarily imply causal associations. Although several classifications are available, a simple approach includes just three types: spurious, indirect, and causal. Spurious associations are the result of selection bias, information bias, and chance.

By contrast, indirect associations (which stem from confounding) are real but not causal. Judgment of cause-effect relations can be tough. Few rules apply, though criteria first suggested by Hill have received the most attention ... (Hill 1965). The only ironclad criterion is temporality: the cause must antedate the effect. However, in many studies, especially with chronic diseases, answering this chicken-egg question can be daunting. Strong associations argue for causation. Whereas weak associations in observational studies can easily be due to bias, large amounts of bias would be necessary to produce strong associations ... Some suggest that relative risks more than 3 in cohort studies, or odds ratios greater than 4 in case-control studies, provide strong support for causation (Sackett et al. 1991). Consistent observation of an association in different populations and with different study designs also lends support to a real effect. For example, results of studies done around the world have consistently shown that oral contraceptives protect against ovarian cancer; a causal relation can, therefore, be argued. Evidence of a biological gradient supports a causal association too. For instance, protection against ovarian cancer is directly related to duration of use of oral contraceptives (Grimes and Economy 1995). The risk of death from lung cancer is linearly related to years of cigarette smoking. In both of these examples, increasing exposure is associated with an increasing biological effect.

Other criteria of Hill's are less useful. Specificity is a weak criterion. With a few exceptions, such as the rabies virus, few exposures lead to only one outcome. Should an association be highly specific, this provides support for causality. However, since many exposures – e.g. cigarette smoke – lead to numerous outcomes, lack of specificity does not argue against causation. Biological plausibility is another weak criterion, limited by our lack of knowledge. 300 years ago, clinicians would have rejected the suggestion that citrus fruits could prevent scurvy or that mosquitoes were linked with blackwater fever. Ancillary biological evidence that is coherent with the association might be helpful. For example, the effect of cigarette smoke on the bronchial epithelium of animals is coherent with an increased risk of cancer in human beings. Finally, experimental evidence is seldom available, and reasoning by analogy has sometimes caused harm. Since thalidomide can cause birth defects, for instance, some lawyers (successfully) argued by analogy that Bendectin (an antiemetic widely used for nausea and vomiting in pregnancy) could also cause birth defects, despite evidence to the contrary (McKeigue *et al.* 1994).

 Activity 5.3

Grimes and Schulz describe the ways that can be used to establish causality. What would be considered to be the strongest evidence?

 Feedback

The authors suggest nine criteria (first suggested by Hill in 1965) by which to evaluate whether an association between two variables is causal. These are:

- Temporal sequence – does the intervention precede the outcome?
- Strength of the association – is there evidence of a strong relationship?
- Consistency of the association – has the association been consistently observed in other studies?
- Biological gradient (dose-response relationship) – does the effect on the outcome increase with increased exposure (or intervention)?
- Specificity of association – is the outcome only found in relation to this exposure (or intervention)?
- Biological plausibility – does the causal relationship make sense?
- Coherence with existing knowledge – does the causal relationship fit in with what is known from the wider literature?
- Experimental evidence – have there been any randomized controlled trials?
- Analogy – is the association similar to others?

Of these criteria, evidence of temporality (where the intervention precedes the outcome), a strong association, consistent observation of the association and a dose-response relationship provide strongest evidence for a causal relationship. The remaining five criteria are weaker.

Summary

Studies evaluating health care should be designed in such a way as to maximize internal validity, by avoiding bias and controlling for confounding. Where the study has been carried out with a highly selected group of patients in a specialized setting, it may be difficult to generalize the results to a wider population. However, it is important to realize that the need to generalize results does not take precedence over the need for internal validity, as invalid results cannot be generalized. Even where a study shows an apparent association between the type of health care and particular health outcomes, it is important to consider the evidence carefully to decide whether this association really represents a causal relationship.

References

Feinstein AR and Horowitz RI (1977) Oestrogen treatment and endometrial carcinoma. *British Medical Journal* 100: 766–7.

Sackett DL (1979) Bias in analytic research. *Journal of Chronic Diseases* 32: 51–63.

Mantel N and Haenszel W (1959) Statistical analysis of the analysis of data from retrospective studies of disease. *Journal of the National Cancer Institute* 22: 719–48.

Grimes DA and Economy KE (1995) Primary prevention of gynaecologic cancers. *American Journal of Obstetrics and Gynecology* 172: 227–35.

McKeigue PM, Lamm SH, Linn S and Kutcher JS (1991) Benedictin and birth defects: 1, a meta-analysis of the epidemiologic studies. *Teratology* 50: 27–37.

Sackett DL, Haynes RB, Guyatt GH and Tugwell P (1991) *Clinical epidemiology: a basic science for clinical medicine*, 2nd edn. Boston, MA: Little, Brown.

Grimes DA and Schulz KF (2002) Bias and causal associations in observational research. *The Lancet* 359: 249–52.

Hennekens C and Buring J (1987) *Epidemiology in medicine*. Boston: Little, Brown.

Hill AB (1965) The environment and disease association or causation. *Proceedings of the Royal Society of Medicine* 58: 295–300.

6

Randomized designs

Overview

This chapter will consider the randomized controlled trial (RCT) as a method of evaluating health care. RCTs involve a deliberate change in the way that existing health care is delivered (e.g. a new treatment) and can be conducted on individuals or communities. You will learn what characterizes an RCT and the challenges of using this method. You will also consider the experience of participating in a trial from the patients' perspective.

Learning objectives

By the end of this chapter you will be better able to:

- **outline the key features and uses of RCTs**
- **explain the methodological limitations of RCTs in health care evaluation**

Key terms

Controls A group of patients that do not receive the treatment that is under investigation.

Double blind When neither patients nor clinicians know the treatment to which patients have been allocated.

Intention to treat analysis When patients' results are analysed on the basis of the study arm to which they were randomly allocated irrespective of the treatment that they actually received.

Placebo An inert medicine or procedure that can be given to the control group in an intervention study.

Randomization The process of allocating patients to treatment based on chance. It is not possible for the investigator, clinician or patient to predict the allocation in advance.

Risk The proportion of individuals experiencing a particular outcome over a specified period of time.

Risk ratio The ratio of the risk of a given outcome from the treatment under investigation to the risk of the same outcome from the control treatment.

Single blind When patients do not know the treatment to which they have been allocated but clinicians do.

Therapeutic equipoise Where the investigator, clinician and patient do not know which of the available interventions is most likely to be beneficial for the patient.

What is an RCT?

An RCT is an experimental study that evaluates a deliberate change in the way that health care is delivered (e.g. a new treatment). Participants are randomly allocated to either a treatment group (sometimes called a treatment arm) or a control group. Patients in the treatment group receive the new treatment whereas patients in the control group might receive either no treatment or the standard treatment. Strict protocols ensure that all other aspects of patients' care are the same for each group. Where possible RCTs should be 'double blind'. That is, neither the investigator nor the patient should know the group to which the patient is randomized. If double blinding is not possible then single blinding should be undertaken. This means that the patient does not know which treatment they have received, but the investigator does. Even when single blinding is not feasible, it should be possible to conceal the treatment allocation. This means that neither the investigator nor the patient know and cannot predict which treatment will be received by the next patient. Allocation concealment can help to avoid selection bias and will be considered in more detail later in this chapter.

RCTs provide rigorous scientific evidence, but randomization can only be undertaken when there is genuine uncertainty (sometimes called 'therapeutic equipoise') about which treatment is most beneficial. Alternative methods for obtaining evidence when RCTs are not appropriate are discussed in the next chapter.

Measures of the effect an intervention

RCTs often measure the risk or rate of a specified dichotomous outcome (e.g. dead or alive, stopped smoking or not; note that the outcome can be either a good or bad event) according to whether an individual received the treatment under investigation. Risk describes the proportion of individuals experiencing the outcome over a known period of time. Usually, an RCT measures the association between the outcome and the experimental treatment by measuring the risk of the outcome over a specified period of time in the group receiving the experimental treatment and dividing this by the risk in the group receiving the standard treatment. This fraction produces a risk ratio. An appropriate test of significance allows you to infer whether the risk ratio differs from unity (i.e. no effect) more than would be expected simply as a result of chance; calculating a confidence interval for the ratio tells you the range within which the true effect is likely to lie. If the risk ratio is greater than 1, the intervention causes an increase in the likelihood of the outcome (providing the RCT is not biased). Conversely, if the risk ratio is less than 1, the intervention causes a decrease in the likelihood of the outcome. You use the significance test and confidence interval to conclude whether the increase/decrease is statistically significant or clinically important.

Rate ratios are calculated and interpreted in the same way as risk ratios. Instead of using risks or rates, some RCTs measure the time taken for participants to experience the particular dichotomous event of interest. These trials are analysed using survival analysis methods, which estimate the relative increase or decrease in likelihood of the outcome as a hazard ratio. The hazard ratio is interpreted in much the same way as a risk ratio.

Note that many RCTs report outcomes that are scaled, or continuously measured (e.g. QoL). In such trials, the effect of the intervention is normally measured by the difference in mean outcome, i.e. the mean outcome for the intervention group minus the mean outcome for the control group.

Pragmatic vs. explanatory trials

RCTs can be either pragmatic or explanatory. Explanatory RCTs measure efficacy and usually require that patients entering the trial be as similar as possible and their treatment to be determined by an agreed protocol. The results may not be very generalizable. Pragmatic RCTs measure effectiveness. They aim to recruit a sample of patients who represent the wider patient population and typical health services, and the treatment they receive is not governed by a protocol.

Randomization

Randomization of participants ensures that selection bias is minimized by preventing systematic differences between the treatment groups. Random allocation means that the group to which the patient is allocated cannot be predicted. The method used to achieve random allocation must therefore be carefully controlled and must not be based on any identifiable characteristic of the participants. If proper randomization is not achieved the internal validity of the trial is threatened. Trials often fail because the methods used for randomization are actually systematic and therefore predictable (Pocock 1983). Appropriate methods for randomization include the use of random numbers tables or computer-generated random numbers, but it is inappropriate to use alternate cases, date of birth, gender or any other identifiable characteristics of patients. These could be used to predict the group to which the patient would be allocated should they join the trial. Investigators could then potentially encourage (or discourage) more of a certain type of patient to participate and potentially influence the results of the trial (Shepperd et al. 1997). Randomization helps to control for unknown confounding factors. It does not guarantee that groups will be equivalent, but makes it *more likely* that they will be equivalent. Lack of equivalence even after randomization is a particular problem in small samples. A sample size of 100 is considered the minimum for randomization to be effective (Elwood 1998).

When the potential confounding factors are known in advance, stratified randomization can be used to achieve equivalence between groups (Shepperd et al. 1997). Randomization is conducted within each factor, for example, if gender is a potential confounding factor then randomization might be conducted separately for men and women, thus ensuring similar numbers of men and women in each group.

The discussion above has focused on randomization of individuals. However, it is also possible to design an RCT to allocate interventions at the group or community level. This is known as 'cluster randomization' and might be necessary for a number of reasons. For example, the intervention is implemented with groups of people rather than individuals; the intervention is delivered to health professionals and the aim is to then investigate the effect on patients; the intervention may be delivered to individuals but inevitably also affects others (i.e. contamination); the intervention concerned with supplying new equipment to an administrative unit (MRC 2002). A new method of purifying water could be evaluated by taking a sample of villages and randomizing them to receive the new water purifier or to continue with the current water source. The outcome might be a change in the rate of diarrhoeal illness in the villages. It is important to note however that control of confounding depends on the number of randomization units rather than the number of individuals within them. Randomization of, for example two or three units (e.g. villages) to each arm of a trial is unlikely to provide sufficient control for confounding factors.

In practice, investigators need to go to some length to ensure that random allocation is achieved, that allocation is concealed and that the procedures are not violated. The precautions that investigators take should be reported in detail in any report of an RCT: 45 per cent of trials reported in general medical journals have been found to be inadequate descriptions of how allocation was concealed (Altman and Dore 1990). Activity 6.1 will help you to think about how random allocation can be achieved, some of the practical difficulties and how these might be overcome.

✎ Activity 6.1

Consider how you might achieve random allocation in an RCT. For example, this might be done by using numbered, sealed envelopes containing the allocated treatment for each participant or numbered containers containing drugs for a drug treatment. Randomization can also be achieved centrally by having field workers ring a dedicated helpline staffed by a statistician who can operate a computer-generated random allocation. Think about the practical difficulties of ensuring that each method is truly random and that the allocation cannot be predicted.

↻ Feedback

Your answers should have considered the points raised in Table 6.1, from Schulz and Grimes (2002). Schulz and Grimes also describe the detail with which these processes need to be reported.

Table 6.1 Minimum and expanded criteria for adequate allocation concealment schemes

Minimum description of adequate allocation concealment scheme	Additional descriptive elements that provide greater assurance of allocation concealment
Sequentially numbered, opaque, sealed envelopes (SNOSE)	Envelopes are opened sequentially only after participant details are written on the envelope. Pressure-sensitive or carbon paper inside the envelope transfers that information to the assignment card (creates an audit trail). Cardboard or aluminium foil inside the envelope renders the envelope impermeable to intense light
Sequentially numbered containers	All of the containers are tamper-proof, equal in weight and similar in appearance
Pharmacy controlled	Indications that the researcher developed, or at least validated, a proper randomization scheme for the pharmacy. Indications that the researchers instructed the pharmacy in proper allocation concealment
Central randomization	The mechanism for contact, e.g. telephone, fax or e-mail – the stringent procedures to ensure enrolment before randomization, and thorough training for those individuals staffing the central randomization office

Source: Schulz and Grimes (2002)

What are the advantages of RCTs?

The main advantage of RCTs is that they maximize internal validity. That is, randomization reduces the likelihood of selection bias and enables the researcher to control for confounding factors more easily. This is why it is so important that randomization procedures are followed properly. Information bias associated with treating one group differently from the other is more or less eliminated by double blinding and is reduced by single blinding. However, in some trials, blinding is impossible. Such trials can still be methodologically rigorous provided that the trial is appropriately designed, randomization is carefully conducted and reported and that investigators adhere to a strict protocol. Information bias associated with recall or inaccurate measurement may still occur in RCTs, though randomization means that this is just as likely to occur in either treatment arm.

An additional advantage of RCTs is that they are the only study design that can control for *unknown* confounding factors. Confounding factors that are already known can be controlled in the design of the RCT, by ensuring that factors such as sex and age are equally represented in each treatment arm. However, unknown confounding factors can only be controlled by randomizing participants to treatment arms. Provided that the sample is large enough, randomization should ensure that the unknown confounding factors are also balanced between the treatment arms.

An RCT based on a strict protocol can therefore provide a precise estimate of a treatment's effects under experimental conditions.

What are the challenges for conducting RCTs?

There are a number of challenges in conducting RCTs. Shepperd *et al.* (1997) provide a useful overview. Their main points are summarized below.

Generalizability (external validity)

Ideally, the participants enrolled in an RCT should represent the total population from which they are drawn and to which the treatment is applicable. If the RCT is not representative, the trial is said to lack generalizability. There are two main reasons why an RCT may suffer from a lack of generalizability. Firstly, inclusion criteria that are too strict may lead to an over-selected group of study participants who do not represent the wider population. While it is necessary to define clear inclusion criteria for each RCT and to document these in the study protocol, they should not be over-prescriptive. Secondly, in some trials, a large proportion of patients refuse to accept randomization. If this group is systematically different from the group that agrees to randomization then the sample on which the trial is conducted may not be representative of the wider population.

Requirement for long-term follow-up

All RCTs require that participants are followed up after the intervention. Most trials lose participants because they have moved away or no longer wish to participate. Some trials have very long follow-up periods, for example trials that evaluate long-term outcomes such as the loosening of hip joints after surgery may require a follow-up period of ten years. These trials are particularly prone to difficulties in retaining cases for follow-up. Activity 6.2 will identify some of the implications of these difficulties and address some possible solutions.

Timing of the trial

There is a relatively short period of time after the introduction of a new therapy during which an RCT can be performed. Immediately after the new therapy has been developed, the level of expertise is relatively low and randomization may be considered unethical on the grounds that it exposes patients to an untested intervention. If a trial is performed at this stage, it may show poor results, reflecting the lack of experience of the clinician. After the therapy has been performed for a while, it may become accepted as the standard, and it may be considered unethical to deny it to patients.

Cost

It is often expensive and time-consuming to design and conduct an RCT. It may require significant changes to working practices, the purchase of new equipment and the training of staff to perform the intervention. It will also be necessary to explain the nature and need for the trial to potential participants and also the need for randomization. When the trial is conducted within the normal health care setting, consultations and procedures will therefore take longer.

Patient and practitioner preferences

In some therapies, a major component is if their beneficial effect is due to the practitioner's or the patient's belief that the patient will get well. Randomization and blinding remove this element. It may be more difficult for patients to have faith in treatments if they do not know what they are receiving and this may reduce the effectiveness of the intervention.

Compliance and crossover bias

Sometimes patients do not comply with the allocated treatment. This may be because they have particular preferences (despite randomization) or because they failed to complete the course (e.g. patients sometimes forget to take medication). Non-compliance is a potential problem for RCTs as it changes the nature of the group receiving treatment.

If patients change therapies during the RCT this is described as 'crossover'. If the patients of one study arm receive less of their allocated treatment, this is described as 'dilution'. If they receive an alternative treatment, this is called 'contamination'. Patients may be changed from one treatment to another because their doctor believes that they are not gaining enough benefit from the initial treatment. While it is proper to act in the best interests of every patient, this may affect the results of the study.

The following extract from Schulz and Grimes (2002) will identify some of the implications of these difficulties and address some possible solutions.

Activity 6.2

Read the following extract by Schulz and Grimes about exclusions and sample size in RCTs. This describes some of the problems that can occur in an RCT when there is a deviation from the protocol, participants drop out, are lost to follow-up or switch treatment. The article discusses how these events can be handled without compromising the scientific integrity of the trial. When you have read the extract imagine that you are conducting a trial of anti-dementia drugs and consider the following questions:

1 Why might cases be excluded prior to randomization? What problems might this present?
2 Why might cases be excluded after randomization? What problems might this present?
3 How can the difficulty of exclusion of cases after randomization be overcome?

Exclusions before randomisation

Investigators can exclude participants before randomisation. The eventual randomised treatment comparison will remain unbiased (good internal validity), irrespective of whether researchers have well-founded or whimsical reasons for exclusion of particular individuals. However, exclusions at this stage can hurt extrapolation, the generalisability, of the results (external validity). For most investigations, we therefore recommend that eligibility criteria be kept to a minimum, in the spirit of the large and simple trial. However, some valid reasons exist for exclusion of certain participants. Individuals could, for example, have a condition for which an intervention is contraindicated, or they could be judged likely to be lost to follow-up. The trial question should guide the approach. Sometimes, however, investigators impose so many eligibility criteria that their trial infers to a population of little apparent interest to anyone, and, in addition, recruitment becomes difficult. If investigators exclude too many participants, or the wrong participants, their results might not represent the people of interest, even though the randomised controlled trial might have been meticulously done – i.e., the results could be true but potentially irrelevant . . .

Exclusions after randomisation

Exclusions made after randomisation threaten to bias treatment comparisons. Randomisation itself configures unbiased comparison groups at baseline. Any erosion, however, over the course of the trial from those initially unbiased groups produces bias, unless, of course, that erosion is random, which is unlikely. Consequently, for the primary analysis, methodologists suggest that results for all patients who are randomly assigned should be analysed, and, furthermore, should be analysed as part of the group to which they were initially assigned. Trialists refer to such an approach as an intent-to-treat analysis. Simply put: once randomised, always analysed as assigned.

Intent-to-treat principles underlie the primary analysis in a randomised controlled trial to avoid biases associated with non-random loss of participants. Investigators can also do secondary analyses, preferably preplanned, based on only those participants, for example, who fully comply with the trial protocol (per protocol) or who receive the treatment irrespective of randomised assignment (on-treatment or as-treated). Secondary analyses are acceptable as long as researchers label them as secondary and non-randomised comparisons.

Discovery of participant ineligibility

In some trials, participants are enrolled and later discovered not to have met the eligibility criteria. Exclusions at this point could seriously bias the results, since discovery is probably not random. For example, participants least responsive to treatment or who have side-effects might draw more attention and, therefore, might be more likely to be judged ineligible than other study participants. Alternatively, a physician who had treatment preferences for certain participants might withdraw individuals from the trial if they were randomly assigned to what he believes to be the wrong group.

Participants discovered to be ineligible should remain in the trial. An exception could be made if establishment of eligibility criteria is difficult. In such instances, investigators could obtain the same information from each patient at time of randomisation and have it centrally reviewed by an outside source, blinded to the assigned treatment. That source, whether a person or group, could then withdraw patients who did not satisfy the eligibility criteria, presumably in an unbiased way.

Postrandomisation, pretreatment outcome

Researchers sometimes report exclusion of participants on the basis of outcomes that happen before treatment has begun or before the treatment could have had an effect. For example, in a clinical trial of a specific drug's effect on death rates, investigators withdrew as non-analysable data on all patients who died after randomisation but before treatment began or before they had received at least 7 days of treatment. This winnowing seems intuitively attractive, because none of the deaths can then be attributable to treatment. But the same argument could be made for excluding data on all patients in a placebo group who died during the entire study interval, because, theoretically, none of these deaths could have been related to treatment. This example illustrates the potential for capriciousness in addressing postrandomisation, pretreatment outcomes.

Randomisation tends to balance the non-attributable deaths in the long run. Any tinkering after randomisation, even if done in the most scientific and impartial manner, cannot improve upon that attribute, but can hurt it. More importantly, this meddling sometimes serves as a post hoc rationale for inappropriate exclusions . . .

Protocol deviations

Deviations from assigned treatment happen in many trials. Some investigators suggest that participants who deviate substantially from the allotted treatment should be excluded in the final analysis, or should be included only up to the point of deviation. Although this approach seems attractive, it has a serious flaw: 'the group which deviates from one protocol and the group which deviates from the other protocol may be so different . . . that the treatment comparison in the remaining patients will be severely biased.' . . . All protocol deviations should be followed up, and their data should be analysed with the group to which they were originally assigned . . . Thus, if researchers report excluding protocol deviates, or if they report moving protocol deviates from one group to another group, the resultant treatment comparison should be considered biased, analogous to an observational study.

Loss to follow-up

Losses to follow-up are perhaps the most vexing of the proffered reasons for exclusions after randomisation. Participants might move or might refuse to continue participating in the trial. Participants lost to follow-up could still be included in the analysis if outcome information could be obtained from another source, such as gathering data from a national death registry. Such opportunities, however, rarely arise. Without outcomes from those lost to follow-up, investigators have little choice but to exclude them from the analysis. Any losses damage internal validity, but differential rates of loss among comparison groups cause major damage. Hence, investigators must minimise their losses to follow-up.

Minimisation of loss in some trials exudes difficulties. Investigators should commit adequate attention and resources to develop and implement procedures to minimise losses. For example, investigators might exclude patients before randomisation if deemed likely to be lost to follow-up. Alternatively, they could obtain contact information to locate lost participants or hire special follow-up personnel who visit unresponsive participants, or both.

Some investigators add innovative twists that cultivate high follow-up rates. One approach uses a large number of conveniently placed follow-up clinics. Too often investigators expect participants to visit a single, inconvenient location. Shortening the data collection instrument to a manageable size caters to the participants' wishes and needs. Investigators foster follow-up by not overburdening participants. Such instruments might not only promote higher follow-up rates, but might also engender higher quality data on the main items of interest. Elimination of loss completely could be impossible, but investigators too frequently profess insurmountable difficulties. Many investigators could work harder than they do to obtain higher follow-up rates.

↻ Feedback

1 Exclusion of some categories of patient before randomization may be necessary. For example, you may want to exclude patients known to have other psychiatric diagnoses. There may also be potential participants whose command of English is insufficient to complete the questionnaire-based outcome measures. You may need to exclude people who are too severe for the drug to be likely to be effective. All of these may be inclusion criteria for your trial. People with dementia may have difficulty with self-report questionnaires and it may therefore be necessary to obtain proxy reports from a carer. Patients without an appropriate carer are unlikely to be able to provide outcome data and you may need to exclude them from your trial. The possible reasons for exclusion prior to randomization should be carefully and clearly documented in the study protocol before beginning recruitment. However, in general the more exclusion criteria that are used, the greater the threat to external validity and generalizability.

2 After randomization, some cases may decide that they no longer wish to receive the treatment to which they were randomized. This may be because they have experienced side-effects of the treatment. This would mean that those experiencing side-effects were unlikely to remain in the trial. Alternatively some people with dementia with particular emotional and/or behavioural symptoms may refuse to participate any more. This could mean that people with particular types of dementia may be excluded from the data. The exclusion of any cases after randomization potentially introduces bias into the comparison of treatment groups and threatens internal validity. The only circumstances under which post-randomization exclusion is not a problem is when exclusion itself is random, but this is very unlikely.

3 The potential bias resulting from exclusion of cases after randomization can be minimized by conducting 'intention to treat' analysis. This means that the primary analysis of the trial is conducted on cases in the groups to which they were originally allocated. Secondary analyses could also be conducted including only those participants who fully comply with the trial protocol (per protocol analysis). However, the nature of these analyses should be specified in advance and should be reported as non-randomized results. Exclusions caused by participants being lost to follow-up can be minimized by strategies such as using follow-up venues that are convenient for the participants, providing efficient follow-up visits that do not overburden the participants, employing someone to coordinate follow up and obtain contact information for each participant that will make follow-up easier.

Designing an RCT

Planning an RCT involves a series of decisions about the particular design of the study, how participants are recruited, adequate sample size and ethical requirements. This section will consider each of these aspects.

In general, RCTs have the advantage of relatively high internal validity (provided randomization procedures are conducted properly, investigators adhere to the study protocol and measurement of outcomes is rigorous). RCTs may also have external validity (provided that the sample can be shown to be representative of the wider population). However, external validity may be threatened by narrow inclusion criteria. Design of an RCT usually consists of a two- or three-parallel group design. A two-parallel group design would compare, for example, drug A with drug B. A three-parallel group design would compare drug A with drug B, with a third group who receive a placebo. There are also other types of RCT. Activity 6.3 below will describe some of the other (less common) types of RCT and help you to consider how they might be used.

All RCTs need to consider how participants are selected. This involves five decisions (Shepperd *et al.* 1997) including: (1) definition of the study population (the type of patient to recruit); (2) developing inclusion criteria (features that patients must have in order to be eligible for the study); (3) developing exclusion criteria (other features that potentially eligible participants must not have); (4) identifying where to recruit patients (this is very much dependent on what the study is about, but could be either hospital-based, such as an outpatient department, or community-based, such as a village clinic); (5) designing a recruitment process to identify eligible participants and invite them to participate in the trial.

All RCTs must also have sufficient sample size and adequate statistical power, discussed in more detail in Chapter 5. In order to calculate sample size it is necessary to know the size of effect that is expected between the two groups. Investigators must therefore have a thorough knowledge and understanding of the existing published literature in the area. Remember that when cluster randomization is planned, the sample size should be large enough to allow sufficient clusters to be included.

All investigators planning an RCT must carefully consider the ethical implications of the study. Many nations have laws or codes of conduct which require that all studies (not just RCTs) are approved by an ethics committee before they can start. This ensures that patients are treated fairly. Most ethics committees will only allow trials to be performed if they follow the principles of the Declaration of Helsinki. In particular, every patient who is recruited to a trial must give informed consent. The purpose of the trial and the relevant procedures must be explained to every participant. Each participant must then sign to say that they have understood all the information that has been explained to them and that they give permission for the investigator to include them in the trial.

There is also a fundamental ethical requirement for all RCTs that a state of therapeutic equipoise exists. This means that there is a genuine uncertainty about which treatment is best. If a state of therapeutic equipoise does not exist then it is unethical to randomize patients to treatments.

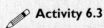 **Activity 6.3**

> The extract below from Shepperd et al. (1997) describes five less common designs of RCT. Read the extract and then describe the advantages and disadvantages that are specific to each type.

Five less common RCT designs

Crossover designs

A crossover design is a design in which each patient receives two or more treatments in sequence and outcomes in the same patient are compared; the comparisons are 'within-patient'. Thus, in a two-treatment, or two-period, crossover study, each patient's response under treatment A is compared with the same patient's response under treatment B, the order of treatments being decided randomly (Senn 1994). In a multi-period crossover design more than two treatments are administered to each patient.

A crossover design is, of course, only applicable when it is possible to treat a patient in more than one way, when the treatment effect is short term, and when the long-term condition of the patient remains fairly stable . . . A crossover design would clearly not be applicable in the comparison of different surgical procedures.

The advantage of a crossover design is that it can produce results that reach a given level of statistical significance with fewer patients. The reason for this is that crossover designs eliminate between-patient variability. However, so as to avoid bias, it is important in the conduct of a crossover design that certain principles are adhered to. These include random allocation of treatment order to each patient (i.e. whether treatment A is administered first or second), consideration of any possible residual effect of the initial treatment on subsequent treatment (carry-over effect), and any possible period effect. A period effect is when the patients tend to respond preferentially to either the first or a subsequent treatment irrespective of what this treatment actually is. For example, the tendency of patients to naturally improve over time (patients tend to present for treatment when their symptoms are most severe) may be reflected in subsequent treatments appearing more effective. A possible carry-over effect can be overcome by the use of a 'wash-out period', an interval between cessation of one treatment and the starting of another. Carry-over effects are residual effects of previous treatments that may influence the participant's response to the current treatment. Wash-out periods are intended to allow sufficient time between successive treatments for the treatment effects to disappear.

n of 1 trials

An n of 1 trial is a randomized double blind crossover comparison of an active drug against placebo in a single patient. This study design can be used by a practitioner to evaluate the effect of a treatment on an individual patient in an unbiased manner . . . Large-scale trials tend to indicate the benefit of treatments 'on average' whereas n of 1 trials indicate the efficacy (or otherwise) of treatments at the level of the individual patient.

Guyatt and colleagues (1986) report using an n of 1 study, using a series of pairs of treatments, to evaluate the effectiveness of a treatment regimen of a patient with uncontrolled asthma. Neither the clinician nor the patient were certain of the effect of two out of the four medications, theophylline and ipratropium, that were part of the patient's treatment regime (although they favoured the theophylline over the ipratropium). The patient agreed to participate in a double blind *n* of 1 trial to evaluate the effectiveness of the two treatments. The patient was first randomized to theophylline or a placebo for a series of 10-day treatment periods, rating his symptoms at the end of each period. After two treatment periods the patient reported feeling much worse at the beginning of each period, the *n* of 1 trial was discontinued and the code broken to reveal that the patient was receiving theophylline at the beginning of each treatment period. This drug was discontinued. The patient then took part in an *n* of 1 trial of ipratropium. A similar procedure was followed and the patient rated his symptoms using an identical scale but on three occasions during a seven-day period. Again after two treatment periods the patient wished the trial 1 to end, reporting an improvement of symptoms at the end of the first treatment period and at the beginning of the second treatment period. When the code was broken it was revealed that the patient was taking ipratropium during these periods. This drug was therefore continued.

Factorial designs

In a factorial design subjects are first randomized to one of the possible treatment groups, and then within each treatment group are further randomized to a different treatment to evaluate a second question. The advantage of this design is that more than one question can be answered in a single trial, without necessarily substantially increasing the costs of the trial . . .

Possible interaction effects between the different treatments should be considered when planning a factorial design. Although it is more likely that a factorial design will identify interaction effects. A factorial design was used for this purpose by (Townsend et al. 1988) to evaluate a hospital discharge scheme. Patients were randomly allocated to standard care or a community-based hospital discharge scheme. The hospital discharge scheme provided elderly patients with the support of a care attendant in their home after discharge from hospital. The care attendants visited the patients before they were discharged, on their first day at home, and for up to 12 hours a week for two weeks. All patients recruited to the study were formally assessed for physical independence and psychological well-being. The study investigators were concerned that the assessment itself would have an effect, perhaps by discovering care needs that would otherwise not be brought to attention. Therefore both the standard aftercare group and the community based hospital discharge scheme were randomly allocated into a further two groups, one group which was assessed at discharge, two weeks and three months and the other group assessed at only three months . . .

Sequential designs

A sequential trial design is a design in which the sample size is not fixed beforehand. Instead, the data are assessed on a large number of occasions, even as frequently as after every new observation, and if any difference between the treatments being compared reaches statistical significance the trial is stopped. The set of criteria for stopping the trial is called the 'stopping rule' . . . A group sequential design is a particular type of sequential design in which only a few interim analyses are performed. This type of design allows the trial investigators to monitor the progress of the trial while keeping the number of inspections low. The advantage of a sequential design is that a statistically significant result may, in principle, be obtained with the minimum number of patients. This clearly is of particular relevance when the condition being treated is life-threatening and ethical issues mean that no more than the minimum number of patients be given an inferior treatment.

There are various factors that need to be taken into account in the conduct and analysis of a sequential design. The 'stopping rule' should ideally relate to only one outcome variable, with other comparisons acting either to confirm or question the results of this one comparison. The main outcome variable should be of sufficiently short time scale, since long-term measures such as mortality would usually not provide information quick enough to prevent any unnecessary entries of patients into the trial. Another factor in devising the stopping rule is that the difference between the treatments must be of clinical significance: statistical significance does not imply clinical significance. It is important that the results of any interim analyses be kept entirely confidential. This is because any trend for one treatment to appear more effective than the other, even if not reaching statistical significance, can make it ethically difficult for those entering patients into the trial to randomize any subsequent patients if they are aware of this fact.

Zelen's design

It is argued that randomization can deter patients from entering trials. Zelen (1979) has proposed an alternative design to overcome some of these potential difficulties. In this design informed consent is obtained after randomization, and only from those patients randomly allocated to the experimental treatment or intervention. Patients who decline the intervention receive the control treatment. In the analysis these patients are grouped with the patients receiving the intervention, and compared with the patients allocated to the control group. If a large number of patients allocated to the intervention cross over to the control group, the study design is compromised, reducing the statistical power. While this type of design may offer an alternative for some trials, it is difficult to implement in many health service research trials where patient outcomes are measured by administering questionnaires, or conducting interviews. In these circumstances patients provide the investigator with a level of information that cannot be collected routinely, but requires active participation from each individual patient. Therefore, when patients consent to participate in a trial they are also consenting to provide detailed information during the follow-up times.

 Feedback

In general the advantages and disadvantages of RCTs described earlier in the chapter also apply to crossover, n of 1, factorial, sequential and Zelen's designs. Shepperd et al. describe additional advantages and disadvantages for each particular design. These are summarized below.

Crossover trials

Advantages – each patient acts as their own control and the between-subject variability is therefore eliminated. Smaller sample sizes are therefore needed.

Disadvantages – there may be a carry-over effect of the first treatment on subsequent treatments. Allowing an interval of time after the first treatment and before beginning the second treatment may help to eliminate this potential source of bias. This is called a 'wash-out' period. Additional bias may occur because patients naturally tend to improve over time. Later treatments may therefore appear to be more effective.

n of 1 trials

Advantages – unlike standard RCTs, n of 1 trials determine effectiveness for the individual rather than the average effectiveness for the group. They can be used in clinical practice to determine the best treatment for an individual patient. *n* of 1 trials are a useful way of using a rigorous scientific method to evaluate a treatment when a standard RCT is not feasible, for example for rare conditions.

Disadvantages – *n* of 1 trials cannot be generalized to any other patients.

Factorial designs
Advantages – participants are randomized first to the treatment and then to a second group (perhaps involving two different ways of administering the treatment). In this way, more than one question can be answered using the same data at little extra cost.

Disadvantages – interaction effects may be present, though these can be exploited to specifically consider the interactions.

Sequential designs
Advantages – enable a statistically significant result to be obtained with the minimum number of patients. This may be particularly important for the evaluation of life-threatening conditions.

Disadvantages – depends on having an appropriate 'stopping rule'. This needs to be described in relation to a single outcome that has a short timescale and must rely on a clinically significant difference between groups rather than simply a statistically signifi-cant difference. It is also necessary to keep the results of interim analyses strictly confidential. Failure to do so would jeopardize the recruitment of additional patients as there would no longer be therapeutic equipoise.

Zelen's design
Advantages – there is less chance that patients will be put off by the prospect of randomization. Arguably this makes more patients willing to take part in the trial.

Disadvantages – this design is difficult to conduct in a health services context as patient consent is only obtained for patients randomized to the intervention group. It therefore relies on routinely-collected data for follow-up (patient consent is required to adminis-ter follow-up questionnaires or interviews). Most health services trials need more sophisticated follow-up data in the form of questionnaires or interviews.

The patient's view of the RCT

The final activity in this chapter will give you the opportunity to think about how an RCT might appear to the patients being asked to take part. This is not an easy exercise, but the feedback will give you some pointers.

Activity 6.4
Imagine that you are asking a patient to take part in an RCT of a new form of treatment for a life-threatening disease. There is an accepted standard treatment which is unlikely to have much success in this case. If the patient agrees to enter the trial, he or she will be randomized to receive either the new treatment or the standard treatment. You

may find this activity easier if you think about a serious disease with which you are familiar. Consider the following questions:

1   How would you describe the principles of an RCT to this patient?
2   Under what circumstances would you be prepared to enter the patient into the study?
3   What might make you decide not to enter this patient?

Feedback

1 The patient needs to know that your treatment will be carried out to the best of your ability. You should make it clear that he or she has the right to refuse to enter the trial, and to withdraw from it at any time, without prejudice to the care received (Mason *et al.* 2002). You need to ensure that the patient understands your diagnosis and prognosis and the likely effects (both beneficial and harmful) of the standard treatment. You should then explain the possible benefits and adverse effects of the new treatment. You might then explain that you are uncertain which treatment would actually turn out to be more effective, and that this study would attempt to find out. The whole purpose of the trial depends on demonstrating whether the benefit of the new treatment exceeds that of the standard therapy. Where the benefit may be small but clinically important, a randomized design is the only reliable way to provide credible evidence that may change the treatment offered to subsequent patients.

You should explain that randomization means that the treatment undertaken is determined by chance. This means that the patients who receive the new therapy will be as similar as possible to those who receive the standard therapy. The allocation may be blinded to ensure that the investigators do not treat patients differently according to the treatment they receive. The patient should also be assured that all information and data will be kept confidentially and will be analysed anonymously.

2 You would have to be certain that neither treatment would be harmful to this particular patient, and that there was no other reason why he or she should not take part in the study. You should not believe that one treatment would be more beneficial than the other, otherwise you would be obliged to provide the better treatment. The patient must understand the nature and purpose of the trial, and give informed consent. The patient must also meet the inclusion criteria for the study.

3 It would not be possible to enter the patient into the trial if there were any reason to believe that it would cause harm – an allergic reaction to one of the treatments, for example. Similarly, you could not enter that patient into the trial if you were not in a state of equipoise (i.e. uncertain as to which treatment was the more effective). The patient should also not be entered into the study if they meet any of the exclusion criteria or fail to meet any of the inclusion criteria.

Meta-analysis

Meta-analysis is a method of combining the results of a number of studies including those that have not been published. Separate meta-analyses could also be conducted of non-randomized studies. Meta-analysis is particularly useful when the results of trials appear to be conflicting or when definitive results have not yet been obtained. Combining the datasets from a number of trials increases statistical power and also enables additional questions to be answered that may not have been posed at the beginning of a particular trial, particularly with respect to generalizability.

Summary

RCTs can be conducted when there is genuine uncertainty about which treatment is most beneficial (therapeutic equipoise). All patients must provide informed consent to take part and ethical approval must be obtained for the study. Patients are allocated to a particular treatment on the basis of chance and the measure of association is the risk ratio. Provided that randomization procedures are followed properly and outcomes are measured rigorously, RCTs tend to have reasonably good internal validity (reduced selection bias and good control of confounding factors). If the sample is also representative of the wider population, they can also have external validity, but this is sometimes threatened by the narrow inclusion criteria. RCTs are often complex to design and expensive to carry out, especially when long-term follow-up is required.

References

Altman DG and Dore CJ (1990) Randomisation and baseline comparisons in clinical trials. *The Lancet* 335: 149–53.

Elwood JM (1998) *Critical appraisal of epidemiological studies and clinical trials*, 2nd edn. Oxford: Oxford University Press.

Guyatt G, Sackett D, Taylor WD, Chong J, Roberts R and Pugsley S (1986) Determining optimal therapy – randomized trials in individual patients. *New England Journal of Medicine* 314: 889–92.

Mason JK *et al.* (2002) *Law and medical ethics*, 6th edn. Oxford: Oxford University Press.

MRC (Medical Research Council) (2002) *Cluster randomised trials: methodological and ethical considerations*, MRC Clinical Trials Series. London: Medical Research Council.

Pocock SJ (1983) *Clinical trials: a practical approach*. New York: John Wiley.

Schulz KF and Grimes DA (2002) Allocation concealment in randomised trials: defending against deciphering. *The Lancet* 359: 614–18.

Senn S (1994). The AB/BA crossovers: past, present and future? *Statistical Methods in Medical Research* 3: 303–24.

Shepperd S, Doll H and Jenkinson C (1997) Randomised controlled trials, in Jenkinson C (ed.) *Assessment and evaluation of health and medical care*. Buckingham: Open University Press.

Townsend J, Piper M, Frank AO, Dyer S, North WR and Meade TW (1988) Reduction in hospital readmission stay of elderly patients by a community based hospital discharge scheme: a randomized controlled trial. *British Medical Journal* 297: 544–7.

Zelen M (1979) A new design for randomized clinical trials. *New England Journal of Medicine* 300: 1242–5.

7 | Non-randomized designs

Overview

When evaluating health care, it is not always possible (or desirable) to perform an experimental study. Instead, non-randomized (observational) study designs can be used to evaluate treatments in the way they are usually administered. In this chapter you will consider the circumstances when RCTs may not be possible.

Learning objectives

By the end of this chapter you should be better able to:

• **outline the key features and uses of non-randomized studies**

Key terms

Non-randomized (observational) A study that examines the effects of health care without influencing the care that is provided or the patients who receive it.

What is meant by a non-randomized (observational) study?

A non-randomized or observational study examines the effects of health care without influencing the care that is provided. Unlike an experimental study it does not require any change in the way that services are delivered. Non-randomized designs assess the naturally occurring variation in health provision. This could be due to differences in practice between practitioners or places at the same time or differences over time within the same place. Variation could be the result of statistical factors (random variation), demand factors on the part of the patient (age/sex of the population, morbidity or patient expectations) or supply factors of the health care (availability of services, clinical judgement). Note however that within social science there is another use for the term 'observational' where it is used to describe a method of systematic watching of behaviour in naturally occurring settings.

The aim of non-randomized studies is to measure the association between variations in process and variation in outcomes. Non-randomized studies can be prospective or retrospective. Where patients and interventions are identified and subsequently followed up to determine outcomes, the study is prospective. If the patients have already received their treatment and experienced the outcome, then the study is retrospective.

Many researchers maintain that experimental studies are the only reliable means of determining the outcome of a medical intervention. The following article by Black (1996) questions this view by highlighting the limitations of experimental studies and the need for observational studies when evaluating health care.

✏ Activity 7.1

Read the article below. Consider the following scenarios (described elsewhere in the article by Black) and for each state briefly why an RCT may not have been the best way to evaluate the effectiveness of health care:

1 A number of trials were conducted on over 3000 patients to evaluate the drug benoxaprofen (Oren) before the drug was launched. The drug was later withdrawn after reports of serious side-effects and a number of deaths. Why would an RCT be an inappropriate method to determine the adverse effects of Oren?
2 It has been suggested that hospitals treating a high volume of patients have better results than those treating a low volume. Why would an RCT be impossible?
3 A trial of glue ear where all the outpatient care and operations were undertaken by senior consultants. Why would an RCT be inadequate?

📖 Experimentation may be unnecessary

When the effect of an intervention is dramatic, the likelihood of unknown confounding factors being important is so small that they can be ignored. There are many well known examples of such interventions: penicillin for bacterial infections; smallpox vaccination; thyroxine in hypothyroidism; vitamin B_{12} replacement; insulin in insulin dependent diabetes; anaesthesia for surgical operations; immobilisation of fractured bones. In all these examples observational studies were adequate to demonstrate effectiveness.

Experimentation may be inappropriate

There are four situations in which randomised trials may be inappropriate. The first is that they are rarely large enough to measure accurately infrequent adverse outcomes. This limitation has been addressed by the establishment, in many countries, of postmarketing surveillance schemes to detect rare adverse effects of drugs ... Huge observational datasets are the only practical means of acquiring such vital information.

A second limitation, also arising from study size, is the difficulty of evaluating interventions designed to prevent rare events. Examples include accident prevention schemes and placing infants supine or on their side to sleep to prevent sudden infant death syndrome. A randomised trial would have needed a few hundred thousand babies.

A third limitation of trials is when the outcomes of interest are far in the future. Three well known examples are the long term consequences of oral contraceptives, which may not be manifest for decades; the use of hormone replacement therapy to prevent femoral fractures; and the loosening of artificial hip joints, for which a 10 to 15 year follow up is needed. The practical difficulties in maintaining such prolonged prospective studies (whether experimental or observational) are considerable, as are their costs. With luck, there will occasionally be times when a randomised trial addressing the question of current interest has already been established decades before and patients from it can then be followed up. Unfortunately such serendipity is all too rare. As a practical alternative to doing nothing, retrospective observational studies can be used to obtain some information on long term outcomes.

Self defeating

Finally, a randomised trial may be inappropriate because the very act of random allocation may reduce the effectiveness of the intervention. This arises when the effectiveness of the intervention depends on the subject's active participation, which, in turn, depends on the subject's beliefs and preferences. As a consequence, the lack of any subsequent difference in outcome between comparison groups may underestimate the benefits of the intervention. For example, it is well recognised that clinical audit is successful in improving the quality of health care only if the clinicians participating have a sense of ownership of the process. Such a 'bottom up' approach is in stark contrast to experimentation, in which the investigator seeks to impose as much control on the subjects in the study as possible – that is, a 'top down' approach. As a consequence, randomised trials of audit might find less benefit than observational studies. The same may be true for many interventions for which clinicians, or patients, or both, have a preference (despite agreeing to random allocation), and where patients need to participate in the intervention – psychotherapy, for example. Many interventions to promote health or prevent disease fall into this category, particularly those based on community development. It is at least as plausible to assume that experimentation reduces the effectiveness of such interventions as to assume, as most researchers have done, that the results of observational studies are wrong.

Experimentation may be impossible

There are some people who believe that any and every intervention can be subjected to a randomised trial, and that those who challenge this have simply not made sufficient effort and are methodologically incompetent. Such a view minimises the impact of seven serious obstacles that researchers have to face all too often. The exact nature of the obstacles will depend on the cultural, political, and social characteristics of the situation and, clearly, therefore, will vary over time.

The first, and most familiar, is the reluctance and refusal of clinicians and other key people to participate. Just because clinical uncertainty, manifest by variation in practice, may exist, this does not mean that each individual clinician is uncertain about how to practise. In 1991 most gynaecologists and urologists in the North Thames region agreed that a randomised trial was needed to investigate the effectiveness of surgery for stress incontinence, but none was prepared to participate as each believed in the correctness of their own practice style. In other words, although 'collective equipoise' existed, 'individual equipoise' was absent. Even when clinicians purport to participate, randomisation may be subverted by clinicians deciphering the assignment sequence.

Ethical objections are a second potential obstacle. It is most unlikely that any ethics committee in an industrialised country would sanction the random allocation of patients to intensive care versus ward care, or cardiac transplantation versus medical management. Observational studies provide an alternative to leaving the question of the effectiveness of these expensive services unevaluated. Furthermore the results of such studies may generate sufficient uncertainty as to make an experimental study acceptable . . .

Political and legal obstacles

Thirdly, there may be political obstacles if those who fund and manage health services do not want their policies studied. In the United Kingdom this was true for general practitioner fund holding and the introduction of an internal market. As a result researchers have been able to perform only a few observational studies, mostly with retrospective controls.

Researchers may also meet legal obstacles to performing a randomised trial. The classic example is the attempt to subject radial keratotomy (an operation to correct short sightedness) to a randomised trial in the United States. The researchers were blocked by private sector ophthalmologists who faced a major loss of income if the procedure was declared 'experimental' because this would have meant that health insurance companies would no longer reimburse them. As a result of legal action, the academic ophthalmologists were forced to declare the operation safe and effective and abandon any attempt at evaluation.

Fortunately, legal obstacles are rare, but a common problem is that some interventions simply cannot be allocated on a random basis. These tend to be questions of how best to organise and deliver an intervention . . .

Contamination and scale

The sixth problem is that of contamination. This can take several forms. If in a trial a clinician is expected to provide care in more than one way, it is possible that each approach will influence the way they provide care to patients in the other arms of the study. Consider, for example, a randomised trial to see if explaining treatments fully to patients, rather than telling them the bare minimum, would achieve better outcomes. This would rely on clinicians being able to change character repeatedly and convincingly. Fortunately there are few Dr Jekylls in clinical practice. Randomisation of clinicians (rather than patients) may sometimes help, though contamination between colleagues may occur, and randomisation of centres requires a much larger study at far greater cost.

The seventh and final reason why it will not always be possible to conduct randomised trials is simply the scale of the task confronting the research community. There are an immense number of health care interventions in use, added to which, most interventions have many components. Consider a simple surgical operation: this entails preoperative tests, anaesthesia, the surgical approach, wound management, postoperative nursing, and discharge practice. And these are just the principal components. It will only ever be practical to subject a limited number of items to experimental evaluation. We therefore need to take advantage of other methods to try and fill in the huge gaps that are always likely to exist in the experimental published findings.

Experimentation may be inadequate

The external validity, or 'generalisability,' of the results of randomised trials is often low . . . The extent to which the results of a trial are generalisable depends on the extent to which the outcome of the intervention is determined by the particular person providing the care. At one extreme the outcome of pharmaceutical treatment is, to a large extent, not affected by the characteristics of the prescribing doctor. The results of drug trials can, in the main, be generalised to other doctors and settings. In contrast, the outcome of activities such as surgery, physiotherapy, psychotherapy, and community nursing may be highly dependent on the characteristics of the provider, setting, and patients. As a consequence, unless care is taken in the design and conduct of a randomised trial, the results may not be generalisable.

There are three reasons why randomised trials in many areas of health care may have low external validity. The first is that the health care professionals who participate may be unrepresentative. They may have a particular interest in the topic or be enthusiasts and innovators. The setting may also be atypical, a teaching hospital for example . . .

Secondly, the patients who participate may be atypical. All trials exclude certain categories of patients. Often the exclusion criteria are so restrictive that the patients who are eligible for inclusion represent only a small proportion of the patients being treated in normal practice. Only 4% of patients currently undergoing coronary revascularisation in the United States would have been eligible for inclusion in the trials that were conducted in the 1970s. It has been suggested that the same problem will limit the usefulness of the . . . randomised controlled trials comparing coronary artery surgery and angioplasty (White 1995). Similar problems occur in trials of cancer treatment. Another facet of this problem is the absence of privately funded patients from almost all randomised trials in the United Kingdom.

The problem of eligibility may be exacerbated by a poor recruitment rate. Although most trials fail to report their recruitment rate, those that do suggest rates are often very low. As little is yet known about the sort of people who are prepared to have their treatment allocated on a random basis, it seems wise to assume that they may differ in important ways from those who decline to take part.

And the third and final problem in generalising the results of randomised trials is that treatment may be atypical. Patients who participate may receive better care, regardless of which arm of the trial they are in.

As a result of these problems, randomised trials generally offer an indication of the efficacy of an intervention rather than its effectiveness in everyday practice. While the latter can be achieved through 'pragmatic' trials which evaluate normal clinical practice, these are rarely undertaken. Most randomised trials are 'explanatory', that is, they provide evidence of what can be achieved in the most favourable circumstances.

The question of external validity has received little attention from those who promote randomised trials as the gold standard. None of the 25 instruments that have been developed to judge the methodological quality of trials includes any consideration of this aspect. The same is true for the guidance provided by the Cochrane Collaboration.

Discussion

Randomised controlled trials occupy a special place in the pantheon of methods for assessing the effectiveness of health care interventions. When appropriate, practical, and ethical, a randomised trial design should be used. I have tried to show that, for all their well known methodological strengths, trials cannot meet all our needs as patients, practitioners, managers, and policy makers. There are situations in which the use of randomised trials is limited either because of problems that derive from their inherent nature or from practical obstacles. While nothing can be done to remedy the former, improvement in the design and execution of trials could, in theory at least, overcome the latter.

Principles versus practice

The problems that could in theory be overcome (and how that could be achieved) include:

- Failure to assess rare outcomes (by mounting large trials with thousands of patients)
- Failure to assess long term outcomes (by continuing to follow up patients for many years)

- Elimination of clinicians' and patients' preferences (by introducing preference arms)
- Refusal by clinicians to participate (by using more acceptable methods of randomisation)
- Ethical objections to randomisation (by exploring alternative less demanding methods of obtaining informed consent)
- Political and legal obstacles (by persuasion)
- The daunting size of the task (by vastly expanding the available funds for experimental studies)
- Overrestrictive patient eligibility criteria (by undertaking pragmatic rather than explanatory trials)

While all the proposed solutions could work in theory, few of them are realistic in practice, presenting as they do enormous problems for researchers and, more importantly, for research funding bodies. For example, it is feasible to randomise tens of thousands of people in a drug trial in which death is the only outcome of interest, but it is unrealistic if more complex and sophisticated outcomes are the relevant endpoints. In many ways the problems that randomised trials encounter arise from a largely uncritical transfer of a well developed scientific method in pharmacological research to the evaluation of other health technologies and to health services.

Several of the other limitations cannot be polarised between principle and practice but are a complex mix of the two. These include:

- Contamination between treatment groups
- The unrepresentativeness of clinicians who volunteer to participate
- Poor patient recruitment rates
- The better care that trial participants receive

In theory all of these could be overcome, although in practice it is hard to see how without the cost of the study becoming astronomical.

Assuming procedural problems could be overcome, two problems of principle inherent in the method would remain. Firstly, the artificiality of a randomised trial probably reduces the placebo element of any intervention. Given that the placebo effect accounts for a large proportion of the effect of many interventions, the results of a trial will inevitably reflect the minimum level of benefit that can be expected. This may be one reason (along with confounding) why experimental studies often yield smaller estimates of treatment effects than studies using observational methods. Secondly, a randomised trial provides information on the value of an intervention shorn of all context, such as patients' beliefs and wishes and clinicians' attitudes and beliefs, despite the fact that such aspects may be crucial to determining the success of the intervention. In contrast, observational methods maintain the integrity of the context in which care is provided. For these two reasons, the notion that information from randomised trials represents a gold standard, while that derived from observational studies is viewed as wrong, may be too simplistic. An alternative perspective is that randomised trials provide an indication of the minimum effect of an intervention whereas observational studies offer an estimate of the maximum effect. If this is so then policymakers need data from both approaches when making decisions about health services, and neither should reign supreme.

Redressing the balance

My intention in focusing on the limitations of trials is not to suggest that observational methods are unproblematic but to redress the balance. The shortcomings of non-experimental approaches have been widely and frequently aired. The principal problem is that their internal validity may be undermined by previously unrecognised confounding factors which may not be evenly distributed between intervention groups. It is currently unclear how serious and how insurmountable a methodological problem this is in practice. While some investigations of this issue have been undertaken, more studies comparing experimental and observational designs are urgently needed.

For too long a false conflict has been created between those who advocate randomised trials in all situations and those who believe observational data provide sufficient evidence. Neither position is helpful. There is no such thing as a perfect method; each method has its strengths and weaknesses. The two approaches should be seen as complementary. After all, experimental methods depend on observational ones to generate clinical uncertainty; generate hypotheses; identify the structures, processes, and outcomes that should be measured in a trial; and help to establish the appropriate sample size for a randomised trial. When trials cannot be conducted, well designed observational methods offer an alternative to doing nothing. They also offer the opportunity to establish high external validity, something that is difficult to achieve in randomised trials.

Instead of advocates of each approach criticising the other method, everyone should be striving for greater rigour in the execution of research, regardless of the method used. 'Every research strategy within a discipline contributes importantly relevant and complementary information to a totality of evidence upon which rational clinical decision-making and public policy can be reliably based. In this context, observational evidence has provided and will continue to make unique and important contributions to this totality of evidence upon which to support a judgement of proof beyond a reasonable doubt in the evaluation of interventions' (Hennekens and Buring 1994).

↻ Feedback

1 In the first example, the RCTs were unlikely to have been large enough to show the occurrence of rare adverse events. Obtaining trial data from samples that were sufficiently large enough to show these effects would be unfeasible and prohibitively expensive. It would therefore have been inappropriate to use RCTs to evaluate this question. Large observational databases (e.g. cohort studies) can provide this kind of data effectively.

2 In the second example, RCTs could in principle help to evaluate the results of high volume vs. low volume hospitals. However, in practice it is very unlikely that patients or clinicians would accept randomization. Few people are likely to support randomly transporting patients to hospitals that are further away. An RCT would therefore be impossible.

3 In the third example, the setting of the RCT is atypical as care is provided by senior consultants whereas it is usually provided by junior medical staff. This means that the generalizability of the results of the trial might be questionable. In this context the RCT might be described as inadequate.

Summary

Black argues strongly that both randomized and non-randomized methods are necessary to the evaluation of health care interventions. He suggests that RCTs have serious limitations and are not always superior to non-randomized studies. The next chapter considers two specific types of non-randomized design: the cohort study and the case-control study.

References

Black N (1996) Why we need observational studies to evaluate the effectiveness of health care. *British Medical Journal* 312: 1215–18.

Hennekens CH and Buring JE (1994) Observational evidence. Doing more good than harm: the evaluation of health care interventions. *Annals of the New York Academy of Sciences* 703: 22.

White HD (1995) Angioplasty versus bypass surgery. *The Lancet* 346: 1174–5.

8 | Cohort and case-control studies

Overview

This chapter will consider two types of non-randomized study design: cohort studies and case-control studies. As with other non-randomized studies, cohort studies do not influence the health care that is provided, and can be used to examine the effect of different systems of delivering care as well as different treatments. This has a number of ethical advantages over an RCT. As randomization is not used in cohort studies, other techniques have been developed to counter the effects of selection bias and confounding variables, and to improve internal validity. The case-control study design is unique because patients are defined as cases or controls on the basis of the *outcome* of their care. They are then investigated to determine which interventions they have received. The study aims to determine whether a statistical association exists between the outcome and the intervention. Case-control studies are largely confined to the evaluation of preventive interventions, such as campaigns to reduce traffic accidents.

Learning objectives

By the end of this chapter you should be better able to:

- **explain the nature and use of cohort and case-control studies**
- **explain the methodological limitations of cohort and case-control studies in health care evaluation**

Key terms

Latency period The time interval between disease occurrence and detection.

Matching A technique used to adjust for the effects of confounding. Controls are selected in such a way that the distribution of potential confounders among the controls is similar to the cases.

Odds ratio The ratio of the odds of exposure in cases to the odds of exposure in controls.

Prospective The patients and interventions (exposures) are identified in the present and followed up in the future to determine the outcomes.

Restriction A technique to reduce the effects of a confounding variable by requiring that all study subjects either have this confounder or do not.

> **Retrospective** The patients have already experienced the interventions (exposures) in the past and are followed up through to the present day.

Cohort studies

Participants in cohort studies are classified according to the exposure to risk factors and followed up to see if they develop the disease in question (Mant and Jenkinson 1997). In the case of health care evaluation patients are classified according to the treatment or intervention they receive, consecutive patients are recruited and the outcomes are measured in terms of health gain. In retrospective cohorts the treatment has already happened by the time of the study. In prospective cohort studies the treatment happens after the cohort has been identified.

Cohort studies compare groups according to the exposure (or treatment) they have received. The groups may be determined internally by dividing a single cohort according to a variable of interest. For example, in a cohort of pregnant women (defined consecutively within a certain geographical area and in a specified period of time) the group who deliver at home could be compared with those who deliver in hospital. Alternatively, the identified cohort could be compared with an external group, for example the general population of a particular country.

A third type of cohort study is known as a 'historically controlled' study (sometimes called a non-parallel cohort study). This type of design uses a combination of retrospective and prospective methods. Historically controlled cohort studies are useful for comparing a new treatment with an existing treatment. The existing treatment is evaluated using a retrospective design. The new treatment is evaluated using a prospective design. The two cohorts are then compared. However, this design is particularly susceptible to confounding and selection bias as different types of patient may be recruited to the retrospective and prospective components. Results may also be influenced by changes in the quality of care over time (irrespective of the actual treatment). This may make the new treatment appear better than it really is.

Measures of the effect of an intervention

Cohort studies measure the same kinds of outcomes as RCTs (dichotomous events, time-to-event data or continuously scaled outcomes; see Chapter 6) so, in principle, exactly the same measures of effects can be calculated, i.e. risk, rate or hazard ratios or differences between mean outcomes for the comparison groups. However, because participants are not randomized to the comparison groups, cohort studies are usually affected by confounding; without randomization, the groups are likely to differ with respect to characteristics that are associated with outcome. The likely presence of confounding means that effects observed in cohort studies should only be considered to represent associations, not causal links. The need for researchers to minimize confounding means that the effect of an intervention on a dichotomous outcome, adjusted for confounding, is almost always reported as an odds ratio rather than a risk ratio. Rate and hazard ratios, and continuously scaled outcomes, can be estimated with adjustment for confounding. As for RCTs, tests of significance should be carried out, and confidence intervals calculated, in order to interpret whether the observed effect estimates could have arisen by chance.

Activity 8.1

Spend a few minutes listing the advantages and disadvantages of cohort studies. It might be helpful to think back over the advantages and disadvantages that were identified for RCTs in the previous chapter and to consider how cohort designs might be similar or different.

Feedback

Advantages – cohort studies are one non-randomized method that can be used to investigate health care as it is provided in every day life and can provide strong evidence that the treatment precedes the outcome (especially in prospective cohorts). Known confounding factors can be statistically controlled.

Disadvantages – As participants are not randomized to treatment, unknown confounding factors cannot be controlled. Selection bias is therefore possible. The possibility of a cohort effect (where a particular cohort is influenced by the historical, economic or social context of that particular era) may limit generalizability. Can be expensive and can take many years to complete (except if retrospective). Retrospective cohorts are dependent on high quality, pre-existing records of both the treatment and outcomes.

Designing a cohort study

Like RCTs, the design of a cohort study involves a series of decisions about how participants are recruited, adequate sample size, ethical requirements and the particular design of the study. Activity 8.2 provides an opportunity for you to design two cohort studies and to consider each of these aspects.

Activity 8.2

Imagine you have been asked to design a cohort study to compare the complication rates of giving birth at home with giving birth in hospital. You will need to consider the intervention that is being compared in the two settings, the inclusion and exclusion criteria, how and when to collect data, how to control for confounding factors and how to analyse the results. Write short notes to describe the steps you would take to design a prospective cohort study and a retrospective cohort study.

↻ **Feedback**

Prospective cohort study

1 Identify the interventions to be compared – the cohorts are defined by these interventions, for example, giving birth at home compared with giving birth in hospital.

2 Define the inclusion criteria – for example, all pregnant women within a particular time period in a certain geographical area.

3 Define exclusion criteria – for example, exclude any women with known medical complications.

4 Enlist support – relevant care workers such as birth attendants, midwives and those in charge of obstetric facilities will need to be involved to help with recruitment and managing follow-up.

5 Invitation to participate – all consecutive patients should be invited to participate.

6 Confounding factors – identify all known confounding factors (e.g. age, parity etc.).

7 Outcomes – choose appropriate outcomes for both mother and infant. Consider the appropriate time frame for outcomes (short- versus long-term). Data collection may be based on routine data, new questionnaires, interviews or a combination.

8 Data collection – identify data collection methods for each confounding factor and each outcome. Data for some confounding factors may be available through routine hospital data, but data on outcomes will generally need to be collected using standardized measures (e.g. questionnaires) specifically for this study.

9 Analysis – compare the outcomes of the two groups after adjusting for known confounding variables. This could be done using a risk ratio.

Retrospective cohort study

1 Identify the interventions to be compared – the cohorts are defined by these interventions, for example, giving birth at home compared with giving birth in hospital.

2 Identify participants who experienced the interventions in the past – for example, all women who gave birth at home or in hospital over a specified period of time and in a certain geographical area.

3 Confounding factors – identify all known confounding factors (e.g. age, co-morbidity, parity etc.). Collect detailed information on these factors for all participants.

4 Outcomes – choose appropriate outcomes for both mother and infant. Consider the appropriate time frame for outcomes (short- versus long-term).

5 Data collection – identify sources of data for each confounding factor and each outcome. Data collection is restricted to routinely available data or ad hoc data. Sources of these types of data are described in more detail in Chapter 3, but could include, for example, hospital episode statistics, insurance claim databases or GP notes. Routine data are limited because they are generally not collected specifically for the study and so may not be exactly the right variable that is needed for the study. Each institution may also have a different method of collecting each variable, making

comparison between institutions difficult. Routine data may also be low quality or incomplete. Ad hoc data are limited as they may not be collected in a standardized or systematic way. Ad hoc data are usually not centralized, so collation can be time consuming.

6 Analysis – compare the outcomes of the two groups after adjusting for known confounding variables. This could be done using a risk ratio.

Ethical concerns

In many countries any form of study (not just RCTs) requires the approval of an ethics committee. The purpose of such a committee is to ensure that participants are treated fairly and without prejudice to their care. It should also ensure that studies are only performed if they seek to provide answers to important clinical problems and there is no unnecessary inconvenience to patients.

Threats to validity

The main threats to validity of a cohort study are similar to those that affect an RCT. However, bias and confounding are potentially more problematic in cohort studies for two reasons. Firstly, cohort studies cannot use randomization to evenly distribute the effects of unknown confounding factors. Secondly, cohort studies cannot blind participants or investigators to the treatment that is received, though investigators can be blinded when analysing the outcomes. This makes it more difficult to eliminate or control potential biases. Activity 8.3 will give you an opportunity to think about the specific ways that biases can affect cohort studies.

 Activity 8.3

You should be familiar with the various forms of bias that can occur in evaluating health care (if you need to refresh your memory, see Chapter 5). Using the example of home versus hospital delivery that you considered in Activity 8.2 again, consider each of the following types of bias and write down an example of each. Try also to think of ways that each type of bias could be minimized in a cohort study.

1 Selection bias.
2 Observation and interviewer bias.
3 Recall bias.
4 Loss to follow-up.

⟳ Feedback

1 *Selection bias*. This could occur if there were some unknown systematic differences between women giving birth at home and those giving birth in hospital. You could control for known potential confounders that might be systematically different between the two groups (e.g. differences in availability of social support, the number of children the woman already has, or social class). However, if there were other confounding variables that were not predicted and were not distributed evenly between the cohorts, selection bias would occur. In a cohort study you cannot randomly allocate patients to receive a particular intervention, but you can measure all known confounders and take any differences between the treatment groups into account in the analyses. By definition, it is not possible to take differences in the distribution of unknown confounders into account in this way.

2 *Observation and interviewer bias*. As observers often cannot be blinded in a cohort study, there is a possibility of observer bias. For example, it is possible that women giving birth in hospital would have better midwifery and medical follow-up. Even if they did not actually receive more intense follow-up, they might receive more monitoring and have more complete records kept of their condition. Observer bias can be reduced by making the data collection procedure as precise and consistent as possible. Investigators should have special training to ensure they ask all participants the same questions in exactly the same way. It may be possible to have study records reviewed and to have patients examined by a 'blinded' investigator. Bias due to the interviewer is also sometimes called 'ascertainment bias'.

3 *Recall bias*. This becomes a problem when the intervention affects how well patients remember the intervention and the outcomes. It is a particular problem with retrospective cohort studies. It is unlikely that there would be errors in recall of major complications such as the need for Caesarean section, but memory of minor adverse outcomes such as a urinary infection may be affected. More recent events might be more easily remembered than those that occurred some time ago. Recall bias is difficult to tackle. Possible strategies to minimize it include ensuring that the interviews take place at the same point in time after delivery for all mothers, and cover the recalled events during the same period of time.

4 *Loss to follow-up*. This is a problem if more patients are lost to follow-up from one cohort than the other. This could occur where hospital patients were only followed up in the hospital, whereas home delivery patients were followed up at home. Mothers who gave birth in hospital might be unlikely to travel a long way back to the hospital just for a follow-up. It is important to make every effort to obtain outcome data from all participants in the study. Loss to follow-up can be reduced by making the follow-up procedure as simple and consistent as possible. For example, it may be more appropriate to visit all mothers in their own homes to assess the rates of complications.

Case-control studies

Case-control studies are different to the types of study that we have considered so far because they define participants on the basis of the *outcome* rather than the intervention. A case-control study starts by defining individuals as cases if they manifest a particular outcome. Controls are then chosen who do not manifest the relevant outcome. The risk factors that are thought to influence the outcome are then compared between cases and controls. The controls should be selected to be as similar to the cases as possible in all other respects. Specific methods of selecting controls are discussed later. Case-control studies are conducted retrospectively. For example, a case-control design could be used to investigate whether eating beef causes CJD. Cases would be defined as those who are diagnosed with CJD and controls would be defined as those not diagnosed. The two groups would be compared in terms of the risk factor of interest (i.e. the proportion of both groups with a diet high in beef).

This design is ideal for investigating rare outcomes where it would take too long to conduct an RCT or a cohort study. Case-control designs also enable several different risk factors to be studied at the same time. However, it is only possible to consider one outcome in a case-control study, because it is the outcome that defines whether a patient is a case or a control.

To help you think about case-control studies, Activity 8.4 uses a hypothetical example to describe the design of a case-control study.

 Activity 8.4

Imagine it has been suggested that vitamin E may reduce the incidence of certain forms of cancer (this is a hypothetical example). You have been asked to design a study to investigate this. You could test this suggestion by randomizing individuals to take vitamin E capsules or not. Alternatively, you could set up a prospective cohort study to compare individuals who happen to be taking vitamin E with others who are not. In either case, you would have to wait many years to discover the effects of vitamin E on cancer incidence. However, a case-control study might be able to provide evidence much more quickly. Consider the following questions:

1 How would you define the cases and controls for this study?
2 How would you define the exposure?
3 What would you expect to find if vitamin E really did provide protection from these forms of cancer?

 Feedback

1 Cases would be people with a diagnosis of one of the relevant forms of cancer. Controls would be individuals without such cancers. After identifying the cases and controls, you would then determine the exposure of cases and controls to the treatment (or risk factor) of interest.

2 The *exposure* in this study would be vitamin E. You would determine the proportion of cases and the proportion of controls who had diets containing high concentrations of vitamin E (or who took vitamin E supplements).

3 If vitamin E is really protective against this cancer, you would expect the cases to show a lower consumption of vitamin E than the controls.

Measures of the effect of an intervention

Case-control studies define case and control groups on the basis of a dichotomous outcome of interest and then compare the relative frequency of the intervention of interest among cases and controls. Cases and controls are sometimes matched on characteristics such as age, gender and the approximate date of intervention. If matched, the data analysis needs to take account of the lack of independence between cases and their matched controls. Groups with and without the intervention are not defined (because subjects are selected on the basis of their outcome) and risks, rates and times to events cannot be calculated meaningfully. The only effect measure that can be estimated directly is the odds ratio. Like cohort studies, case-control studies are usually affected by confounding. Therefore, effects observed in such studies should only be considered to represent associations, not causal links. Tests of significance should be carried out, and confidence intervals calculated, in order to interpret whether the observed effect estimates could have arisen by chance.

Advantages of the case-control study

The case-control study is seldom used to evaluate health care. However, there are a few circumstances where it has a number of advantages over other designs.

Rare adverse outcomes

As the cases are defined by their having experienced the outcome of interest, it is possible to investigate adverse outcomes that are rare, such as deaths following straightforward surgery for benign conditions, or mental impairment following whooping cough vaccination.

Speed and low costs

Case-control studies are often cheaper and easier to perform than other types of design. This is largely because the case-control study is a form of retrospective study. The outcome has already occurred and there is no need to wait for patients to experience it.

Ethical issues

Assessment of the ethical implications of case-control studies is relatively straight-forward. Case-control studies are retrospective and do not involve any changes to the treatment that patients receive, so they do not influence the outcomes at all. However, it is still necessary to ensure that participants are treated fairly and to obtain the approval of an ethics committee before obtaining patient data or administering questionnaires or interviews.

Disadvantages of the case-control study

Bias

Case-control studies are particularly prone to selection bias because the controls are selected rather than random or consecutive. Two techniques for reducing this bias are 'matching' of controls and 'restricting' of the sample. These are discussed below. As with all retrospective studies, data collection may also be subject to recall bias. Although it is not possible to eliminate recall bias, measuring outcomes in the same way in both case and control groups ensures that its effect is similar in both groups.

Causal uncertainty

Prospective studies can usually determine that interventions occur before out-comes. However, this may not be the case with case-control studies, where the outcome is identified first. If the outcome is a disease with a long latent period, it may be possible that the disease predated the intervention.

Threats to validity

Case-control studies suffer from similar problems of bias and confounding as cohort studies. You have already read about confounding, bias and chance in Chapter 5. However, these are such important subjects that it is worth considering some examples of the way that they can affect case-control studies.

The most important source of bias in the design of case-control studies is selection bias. Ideally, controls and cases should be identical in every way except the outcome of interest and the exposure that causes this outcome. However, it is quite possible that the likelihood of an individual's being selected as a case or control might be affected by whether this individual was exposed to the risk factor of interest. Selection of appropriate controls is therefore one of the most important aspects of designing a case-control study. Where the cases are hospital patients, it is sometimes necessary to select controls from hospital patients suffering from different diseases. However, the difference in diagnoses can produce confounding.

The next extract will illustrate some of these problems and outline two ways in which confounding can be minimized.

 Activity 8.5

Read the extract below from Mant and Jenkinson (1997). Think again about the hypothetical example you considered in Activity 8.4 (a case-control study to investigate whether vitamin E reduces the incidence of certain forms of cancer). Describe how you could use each of the following techniques to reduce the effect of confounding:

1 Restriction.
2 Matching.

 Confounding

A *confounding* factor is something that is associated both with the exposure and the disease being investigated. For example, there have been a number of case control studies looking at whether taking the oral contraceptive pill (ocp) might be linked to an increased risk of breast cancer. A meta-analysis . . . of these studies concluded that women who take the oral contraceptive pill are at increased risk of having breast cancer diagnosed (Collaborative Group on Hormonal Factors in Breast Cancer 1996). However, it has been suggested that the observed association may be due to confounding: Hemminki (1996) argues that women who take oral contraceptives are more likely to be fertile and be sexually active than women not on the pill. If either fertility or sexual activity was related to breast cancer risk, then an observed association between the ocp and breast cancer may have nothing to do with a harmful effect of the pill, but simply reflect the differing fertility or sexual activity of people who take the pill compared to non-users.

It has also been argued that another possible confounder of any relationship between the ocp and breast cancer might be cigarette smoking (Trichopoulos and Katsouyanni 1989). Commenting on one of the case control studies (UK National Case-Control Study Group 1989), Trichopoulos and Katsouyanni argue that women who use the ocp are advised not to smoke, and therefore smoking could be a confounder if it protects against breast cancer. In other words, if women give up smoking to be on the ocp, they may inadvertently be increasing their risk of breast cancer by losing the (postulated) protective effect of tobacco. In fact, recent evidence suggests that smoking increases rather than reduces the risk of breast cancer (Bennicke et al. 1995; Morabia et al. 1996). If this is the case, then confounding would still be occurring, but the effect of smoking would be to mask any link between the ocp and breast cancer, if indeed people who take the ocp are less likely to smoke. In other words, confounding can work in both directions: it may cause an apparent relationship between a risk factor and a disease that does not in fact exist, or it may cause a real association to disappear. The possibility of confounding can be taken into account in the design and in the analysis of a case control study.

In the design of the study one could *restrict* the selection of cases and controls in a way that would nullify the effects of the confounder. For example, one could remove the possibility of smoking confounding the effects of the ocp on risk of breast cancer by only selecting cases and controls who did not smoke. Alternatively, one could select the controls in such a way that they *matched* the cases with regard to the presence or absence of the risk factor.

In this example, a case (of breast cancer) who was a smoker would need to be matched with a control (someone who does not have breast cancer) who also smokes. It is quite common for the controls in a case control study to be matched to the cases with regard to a couple of potential confounders, particularly age and sex.

However, in a matched study one cannot look at the impact of the matched variable(s) on the risk of disease, and if one 'overmatches' then one may mask the true effect of the risk factor(s) that are being investigated. If one has used a matched design, it is important that the analysis takes account of the matching. In Blair *et al.*'s (1996) study of cot death, the controls were selected from the same neighbourhood and were the same age as the infants who had died. This matching necessitates a slightly more sophisticated derivation of the odds ratio . . .

 Feedback

1 Restriction is used to avoid the effects of a confounding factor by ensuring that patients in each study group (i.e. cases and controls) are affected in the same way by this confounder. If smoking is the confounding variable, the study could be restricted to include only smokers or non-smokers. In this way both cases and controls would be similar with regard to smoking.

2 Matching is another technique to avoid the effect of a confounding variable. Each case is matched with a particular control with regard to the presence of the confounder. For example, each case who smokes would be matched with a control who smokes a similar amount. Each non-smoking case would be matched with a non-smoking control.

Summary

Observational studies utilize naturally occurring variation and can be useful for evaluating health care in exactly the way that it is delivered. They may be the only method of evaluating interventions for which randomization is not appropriate.

You have now considered two types of observational design: cohort designs and case-control designs. In cohort studies participants are identified on the basis of the intervention and are followed up to determine the proportion (or rate) of specified outcomes in each cohort. Cohort studies can be either retrospective or prospective. Internal validity of the cohort study is potentially threatened by the same factors as in an RCT. However, randomization cannot be used to avoid selection bias and the influence of confounding factors, so it is necessary to measure and adjust for all known confounding factors. The measure of association is the risk ratio.

The case-control study is a retrospective design where participants are identified on the basis of the outcome. Controls are chosen to be as similar as possible to cases on all other variables. Case-control studies are rarely used in health care evaluation, but are sometimes useful for evaluating adverse events or rare conditions. They are relatively quick and cheap to conduct, but are particularly prone to bias. Selection bias is reduced by careful selection of controls and confounding may be reduced by restricting the sample or matching cases and controls. The measure of association is the odds ratio.

References

Bennicke K, Conrad C, Sabroe S and Sorensen HT (1995) Cigarette smoking and breast cancer. *British Medical Journal* 310: 1431–3.

Blair PS, Fleming PJ, Bensley D *et al.* (1996) Smoking and sudden infant death syndrome. *British Medical Journal* 313: 195–8.

Collaborative Group on Hormonal Factors in Breast Cancer (1996) Breast cancer and hormonal contraceptives: collaborative reanalysis of individual data on 53,297 women with breast cancer and 100,329 women without breast cancer from 54 epidemiological studies. *The Lancet* 347: 1713–27.

Doll R, Peto R, Wheatley K, Gray R and Sutherland I (1994) Mortality in relation to smoking: 40 years' observations on male British doctors. *British Medical Journal* 309: 901–11.

Hemminki E (1996) Oral contraceptives and breast cancer. *British Medical Journal* 313: 63–4.

Mant J and Jenkinson C (1997) Case-control and cohort studies, in Jenkinson C (ed.) *Assessment and evaluation of health and medical care.* Buckingham: Open University Press.

Morabia A, Bernstein M, Heritier S and Khatchatrian N (1996) Relation of breast cancer with passive and active exposure to tobacco smoke. *American Journal of Epidemiology* 143: 918–28.

Trichopoulos D and Katsouyanni K (1989) Oral contraceptives, tobacco smoking and breast cancer risk. *The Lancet* II: 158.

UK National Case-Control Study Group (1989) Oral contraceptive use and breast cancer risk in young women. *The Lancet* I: 973–82.

9 | Ecological designs

Overview

All the evaluation study designs considered so far have measured both intervention and outcome at the level of the individual. Ecological studies make at least one of these measurements at the level of groups instead of individuals. This session will introduce you to the principles of ecological studies and describe some of the circumstances where they may be useful. It will also consider some of the main threats to the validity of ecological studies.

Learning objectives

By the end of this chapter you should be better able to:

- **outline uses and key features of ecological studies in health care evaluation**
- **explain time-series analysis**
- **describe the advantages and limitations of ecological designs**

Key terms

Cross-sectional study Study design where exposure and outcome are measured at the same time.

Ecological fallacy The effects measured in groups may not be applicable at the level of individuals.

Multiple groups Measurements of exposure and outcome are made on a number of groups at a single point in time.

Multiple time-series A number of different groups are defined and measurements made at a number of points in time.

Single time-series One group (or population) is defined and measurements are made at a number of points in time.

What is an ecological study?

Ecological studies use data from the population rather than the individual. Unlike the other designs that you have considered, no attempt is made to identify individuals receiving health care or to relate interventions to outcomes for individuals. Ecological studies have been used for many different purposes in health services research. Some examples include studies to investigate international differences in infant mortality, the correlation between alcohol consumption and traffic accidents, staffing levels of health centres and vaccination rates and equity of access to care between regions. Data from different countries or regions can be compared at the same time. Alternatively, data from the same country or region at different times can be compared.

The data in ecological studies do not give any indication of how individuals vary within the group or whether any variation is similar in different groups. Ecological studies are also often conducted using data that has been collected for another purpose. Data on alternative explanatory factors may not be available.

Activity 9.1

Imagine you have designed an ecological study to determine the extent to which practice changed after the issue of a national guideline on the use of Alzheimer's drugs. You might have routine data from the whole country on the overall use of drugs before the guideline was issued and after it was issued. The pattern over time might be similar to Figure 9.1.

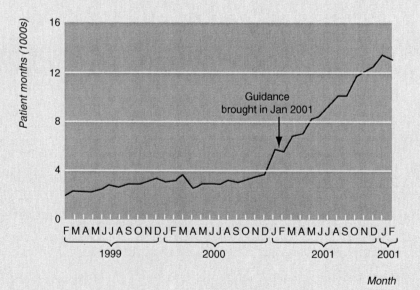

Figure 9.1 Total use of Alzheimer's drugs in the community

Source: Sheldon *et al.* 2004

1   Describe the conclusions you would be able to draw from these data.
2   What are the limitations to the conclusions you are able to draw?

↻ Feedback

1   You would be able to conclude that there was a general upward trend just before the guidelines were issued.

2   You would not be able to make any conclusions about other factors that might explain this finding. In addition, the data do not reveal anything about the prescribing practice of individual GPs who were part of the study. To illustrate, consider the following sets of data. Groups A and B below both have the same mean age, but their age structures are quite different. If these data were compared the means of the two populations are identical. The analysis would not reveal that they were in fact different at the individual level.

Group A
Individual age (years):

1   31
2   27
3   38
4   35
5   37

Mean age = 33.6

Group B
Individual age (years):

1   14
2   61
3   12
4   15
5   66

Mean age = 33.6

Advantages of ecological studies

- Ecological studies may be able to produce results for little cost by taking advantage of routine data sources. They can also exploit natural variations between groups or between different time periods (e.g. the introduction of a new intervention).
- Ecological studies may be the only feasible way of evaluating the effects of health care programmes where data on individuals' outcomes are not available.
- Ecological studies provide the appropriate strategy for assessing changes in

legislation or health policies, such as health promotion campaigns, that are aimed at groups.

- Ecological studies can be useful for generating hypotheses that can then be investigated at the individual level.

Disadvantages of ecological studies

While ecological studies provide a useful means of studying the effects of an exposure on groups, they do have some major drawbacks too. The main disadvantage is the 'ecological fallacy' (or ecological bias). This is where the effects measured on groups may not always be applicable at the individual level. For example, if a population receives a new, easily accessible health centre, the health of the population may improve. However, the improvement may not actually occur in the people who attend the new health centre. Therefore, the improvement may be falsely attributed to the new facility.

Different types of ecological study: time-series

There are several different types of ecological study. One of the most common is a time-series design which involves collecting data before and after an intervention and comparison with a parallel control group. However, this is only one type of ecological design. Activity 9.2 describes three types of design: multiple group analysis, single time-series (time-trend) and multiple time-series (mixed study).

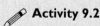 **Activity 9.2**

Read the extract below by Morgenstern (1995) which describes in detail the design of ecological studies and then briefly summarize each type of design. The article is based on examples about aetiology (study of causes of diseases) rather than health care evaluation. However, the principles are the same.

 Ecologic studies in epidemiology: concepts, principles, and methods

Study designs

In an ecologic study design, the planned unit of analysis is the group. Ecologic designs may be classified on two dimensions: the method of exposure measurement and the method of grouping (Kleinbaum et al. 1982; Morgenstern 1982). Regarding the first dimension, an ecologic design is called *exploratory* if the primary exposure of potential interest is not measured, and *analytic* if the primary exposure variable is measured and included in the analysis. In practice, this dimension is a continuum, since most ecologic studies are not conducted to test a single hypothesis. Regarding the second dimension, the groups of an ecologic study may be identified by place (multiple-group design), by time (time-trend design), or by a combination of place and time (mixed design).

Multiple-group study

EXPLORATORY In this type of exploratory study, we compare the rate of disease among many regions during the same period. The purpose is to search for spatial patterns that might suggest an environmental etiology or more specific etiologic hypotheses. For example, the National Cancer Institute (NCI) mapped the age-adjusted cancer mortality rates in the U.S. by county for the period 1950–69 (Mason *et al*. 1975). For oral cancers, they found a striking difference in geographic patterns by sex: among men, the mortality rates were greatest in the urban North-east, but among women, the rates were greatest in the South-east. These findings led to the hypothesis that snuff dipping, which is common among rural southern women, is a risk factor for oral cancers (Blot and Fraumeni 1977). The results of a subsequent case-control study supported this hypothesis (Winn *et al*. 1981) . . .

In mapping studies, such as the NCI investigation, a simple comparison of rates across regions is often complicated by two statistical problems. First, regions with smaller numbers of observed cases show greater variability in the estimated rate; thus the most extreme rates tend to be observed for those regions with the fewest cases. Second, nearby regions tend to have more similar rates than do distant regions (i.e. autocorrelation) because unmeasured risk factors tend to cluster in space. Statistical methods for dealing with both problems have been developed by fitting the data to an autoregressive spatial model and using empirical Bayes techniques to estimate the smoothed rate for each region (Clayton and Kaldor 1987; Mollie and Richardson 1991; Moulton *et al*. 1994) . . .

ANALYTIC In this type of study, we assess the ecologic association between the average exposure level or prevalence and the rate of disease among many groups. This is the most common ecologic design; typically, the unit of analysis is a geopolitical region. For example, Hatch and Susser (Hatch and Susser 1990) examined the association between background gamma radiation and the incidence of childhood cancers between 1975 and 1985 in the region surrounding a nuclear power plant. Average radiation levels for each of 69 tracts in the region were estimated from a 1976 aerial survey. The authors found positive associations between radiation level and the incidence of leukemia (an expected finding) as well as solid tumors (an unexpected finding).

Data analysis in this type of multiple-group study usually involves fitting the data to a mathematical model . . .

Time-trend study

EXPLORATORY An exploratory time-trend or time-series study involves a comparison of the disease rates over time in one geographically defined population. In addition to providing graphical displays of temporal trends, time-series data can also be used to forecast future rates and trends. This latter application, which is more common in the social sciences than in epidemiology, usually involves fitting the outcome data to autoregressive integrated moving average (ARIMA) models (Helfenstein 1991; Ostrom 1990) . . .

A special type of exploratory time-trend analysis often used by epidemiologists is age-period-cohort (or cohort) analysis. Through graphical displays or formal modeling techniques, the objective of this approach is to estimate the separate effects of three time-dependent variables on the rate of disease: age, period (calendar time), and birth cohort (year of birth) (Holford 1991; Kleinbaum *et al*. 1982). Because of the linear dependency of these three variables, there is an inherent statistical limitation (identification problem) with the interpretation of age-period-cohort results. The problem is that each data set has alternative explanations with respect to the combination of age, period, and cohort effects; there is no unique set of effect parameters when all three variables are considered simultaneously. The only way to decide which interpretation should be accepted is to consider the findings in light of prior knowledge and, possibly, to constrain the model by ignoring one effect . . .

ANALYTIC In this type of time-trend study, we assess the ecologic association between change in average exposure level or prevalence and change in disease rate in one geographically defined population. As with exploratory designs, this type of assessment can be done by simple graphical displays or by time-series regression modeling (e.g. Ostrom 1990). With either approach, however, the interpretation of findings is often complicated by two problems. First, changes in disease classification and diagnostic criteria can produce very misleading results. Second, the latency of the disease with respect to the primary exposure may be long, variable across cases, or simply unknown . . .

Mixed study

EXPLORATORY The mixed ecologic design combines the basic features of the multiple-group study and the time-trend study. Time-series (ARIMA) modelling or age-period-cohort analysis can be used to describe or predict trends in the disease rate for multiple populations . . .

ANALYTIC In this type of mixed ecologic design, we assess the association between change in average exposure level or prevalence and change in disease rate among many groups. Thus the interpretation of estimated effects is enhanced because two types of comparisons are made simultaneously: change over time within groups and differences among groups . . .

 Feedback

Multiple group analysis
The rate of disease is measured in a number of different groups (or populations) during the same period of time. This design can be used to identify spatial patterns of disease, for example the prevalence of childhood cancer near a nuclear power plant.

Single time-series analysis (time-trend)
One group (or population) is defined and measurements are made at a number of points in time. For example, the simplest time-series design would compare outcomes before and after an intervention, though a larger number of time points would be preferable.

Multiple time-series analysis (mixed study)
A number of different groups are defined and measurements made at a number of points in time. This allows trends in disease rates to be monitored for multiple populations. For example, investigating the association between changes in the hardness of the water supply in several different areas with mortality from cardiovascular disease.

Activity 9.3

Imagine a country has been collecting routine data on perinatal mortality for many decades. In 2005 a new programme of mother-child health care was introduced which was intended to substantially improve antenatal care. An ecological study could be used to evaluate this intervention by using a time-series design.

1   Describe how you could use a time-series design to evaluate this intervention.

Now imagine that a change in trend is observed after the intervention. Perinatal mortality is declining faster than before the introduction of the new scheme.

2   What are the difficulties in interpreting this finding?

Feedback

1   The simplest design is to compare the outcome before and after the intervention. The outcome, perinatal mortality, is measured at one point in time before and at one point in time after the new intervention has been introduced (though you would probably prefer to look at a larger series of observations and analyse changes in trend of perinatal mortality after the intervention). In identifying the pattern of change, you could analyse the slope of the trend curve – before and after the intervention – and measure the decline in perinatal mortality in percentage terms.

2   A major problem of the time-series design is in identifying an attribution between outcomes and intervention. Is the observed decline in mortality really attributable to the improvement of pre-natal services? Answering this question is particularly difficult when:

- there are *concurrent interventions* that could also change the outcome (e.g. a health education campaign, change in child benefit)
- the intervention to be evaluated is *diffuse* (e.g. if the new programme were phased in over a long period of time it would then be more difficult to identify an effect)
- the intervention to be evaluated has a long *latent period*; this is the case when there is a long period of time between the intervention and the effect (e.g. changes in tobacco legislation and the decline in lung cancer mortality)

There are other practical difficulties with time-series data related to the *estimation* of the effect, such as the following:

- *bias* – due to changes in classification, for example, or the way data are collected
- *noise* – this is the variation of single observations around the underlying trend; some observations lie above and some below the trend line and changes in one direction could be mistaken for a change in trend, if the observation period is too short
- *cycles* – temporal changes of the outcomes (day-to-day, or season to season) are not uncommon and need to be controlled for when estimating the effect of an intervention (such as seasonal changes in the incidence of infectious diseases)

It may be of interest to you that a number of mathematical models have been developed to reduce errors in effect estimation.

Summary

Ecological studies measure outcomes at the level of groups rather than that of the individual. They use routine data to provide a quick, relatively cheap estimate of association. When data in individual outcomes are not available, these studies may be the only feasible way of evaluating the effects of health care programmes. Ecological studies can also be useful for generating hypotheses to be investigated at the individual level. However, ecological studies have difficulty establishing causality because they cannot link outcome to exposure at the individual level (ecological fallacy). The time-series design allows examination of group-level variations over time. Problems of using this design in health care evaluation are related to assessing the magnitude of the effect and attributing it to the intervention.

References

Blot WJ and Fraumeni JF Jr. (1977) Geographic patterns of oral cancer in the United States: etiologic implications. *Journal of Chronic Diseases* 30: 745–57.

Clayton D and Kaldor J (1987) Empirical Bayes estimates of age standardized relative risks for use in disease mapping. *Biometrics* 43: 671–81.

Hatch M and Susser M (1990) Background gamma radiation and childhood cancers within ten miles of a US nuclear plant. *International Journal of Epidemiology* 19: 546–52.

Helfenstein U (1991) The use of transfer function models, intervention analysis and related time series methods in epidemiology. *International Journal of Epidemiology* 20: 808–15.

Holford TR (1991) Understanding the effects of age, period, and cohort on incidence and mortality rates. *Annual Review of Public Health* 12: 425–57.

Kleinbaum Dg, Kupper LL and Morgenstern H (1982) *Epidemiologic research: principles and quantitative methods*. New York:Van Nostrand Reinhold.

Mason TJ, McKay FW, Hoover R, Blot WJ and Fraumeni JF Jr. (1975) Atlas of cancer mortality for US counties:1950–1969. *DHEW* Publ. No. (NIH) 75–780. Washington, DC: US GPO.

Mollie A and Richardson S (1991) Empirical Bayes estimation of cancer mortality rates using spatial models. *Statistics in Medicine* 10: 95–112.

Morgenstern H (1982) Uses of ecologic analysis in epidemiologic research. *American Journal of Public Health* 72: 1336–44.

Morgenstern H (1995) Ecologic studies in epidemiology: concepts, principles and methods. *Annual Review of Public Health* 16: 61–81.

Moulton LH, Foxman B, Wolfe RA and Port FK (1994) Potential pitfalls in interpreting maps of stabilized rates. *Epidemiology* 5: 297–301.

Ostrom CW Jr (1990) *Times series analysis: regression techniques*, 2nd edn. Newbury Park, CA: Sage.

Sheldon, TA *et al.* (2004) What's the evidence that NICE has been implemented? *British Medical Journal*, 329: 999.

Winn DM, Blot WJ, Shy CM, Pickle LW, Toledo A and Fraumeni JF Jr. (1981) Snuff dipping and oral cancer among women in the southern United States. *New England Journal of Medicine* 304: 745–9.

Comparing study designs

Overview

This chapter provides an opportunity to revise what you have learned so far about study design. You have already examined RCTs, cohort studies, case-control studies and ecological studies. When evaluating the effectiveness of a health care intervention, you need to choose which design is most appropriate. In this chapter you will revise the advantages and disadvantages of each design and consider the situations in which you would choose one design over the others.

Learning objectives

By the end of this chapter you should be better able to:

- **compare critically the validity of designs used in the evaluation of health care**
- **make an informed choice of appropriate study designs to evaluate the effectiveness of different interventions**

Advantages and disadvantages of study designs

You have already considered the strengths of each type of study design, but you have not yet explicitly compared study designs in terms of how they might be used. This chapter will, first, review the strengths and weakness of each type of study, then illustrate their practical uses.

 Activity 10.1

Briefly describe the nature of an RCT, its advantages and disadvantages.

 Feedback

In this design, participants are assigned to an intervention (or treatment) in such a way that nobody can predict who will receive any given intervention. Follow-up is prospective. The measure of association is the risk ratio (although it is possible to use the odds ratio).

Advantages

1 It is possible to measure the incidence of relevant outcomes.

2 An RCT is particularly effective at avoiding selection bias and confounding.

3 It is the only design that can reduce the effect of unknown confounders.

4 Prospective follow-up allows outcomes to be measured in terms of incidence.

5 Multiple outcomes can be measured.

Disadvantages

1 RCTs are time-consuming and expensive to design and undertake.

2 The design and analysis can be complex, particularly if it involves randomizing groups rather than individuals.

3 There may be ethical difficulties. In particular an RCT can only be undertaken if therapeutic equipoise exists.

4 Subjects may be quite different from the wider patient population, leading to difficulties in generalizing the results.

5 Losses to follow-up can cause serious bias.

 ## Activity 10.2

Briefly describe the nature of a cohort study, its advantages and disadvantages.

 ## Feedback

In this design, groups of individuals are defined according to the health care interventions that they are receiving. Studies may be prospective or retrospective. Retrospective cohort studies define groups according to their past interventions. This means that there has been time for outcomes to develop. In contrast, prospective cohorts define groups according to future or current interventions. The measure of association is the risk ratio (although it is possible to use the odds ratio).

Advantages

1 It is possible to measure the incidence of relevant outcomes.

2 The time sequence of intervention and outcome can be measured, which makes it easier to determine causality.

3 Unusual interventions or rare exposures can be studied if large cohorts are assembled.

4 Multiple outcomes can be studied for any one exposure.

5 Retrospective cohort studies can produce relatively quick results on long-term outcomes.

Disadvantages

1 Retrospective cohort studies may have difficulty identifying the intervention precisely.

2 Losses to follow-up can cause serious bias.

3 Observation bias can be a problem.

4 There is no mechanism to deal with unknown confounders.

 Activity 10.3

Briefly describe the nature of a case-control study, its advantages and disadvantages.

 Feedback

Although this design is rarely used in health care evaluation, it can be useful for evaluating rare exposures. The design starts by identifying individuals (cases) who have the health outcome of interest. Controls are selected and the exposure status of cases and controls is compared. The measure of association is the odds ratio. It is not possible to calculate risk ratios.

Advantages

1 It is possible to investigate multiple exposures.

2 As this is a retrospective design, results may be obtained relatively quickly.

3 Case-control studies are very useful for studying rare outcomes.

Disadvantages

1 Selection bias is a major problem because the controls are chosen by the investigator. It is important to choose controls in such a way as to minimize confounding.

2 Observation and recall bias are also major problems.

3 Case-control studies are not good at investigating rare exposures.

4 Only one outcome can be studied (as the outcome is used to define cases).

5 It is difficult to determine the time sequence of exposure and outcome, making it more difficult to determine causality.

6 Case-control studies cannot measure incidence.

 Activity 10.4

Briefly describe the nature of an ecological study, its advantages and disadvantages.

Feedback

Either the intervention or the outcome, or both, are measured at the level of groups or populations rather than at individual level. Ecological studies aim to investigate differences in outcome between groups having different exposures (multiple group studies). Alternatively, they may evaluate the change in outcome over time in one or more groups (time-series studies). The measure of association is often expressed as an odds ratio or in terms of a correlation coefficient.

Advantages
1 Ecological studies are usually relatively cheap and easy to design.

2 Results may be obtained quickly in multiple group studies.

3 They are useful in generating hypotheses for further investigation.

4 Appropriate mathematical modelling can be used to investigate outcomes and exposures that show a variety of trends over time.

Disadvantages
1 Multiple group studies can only measure prevalence, not incidence.

2 The ecological fallacy limits the ability of ecological studies to determine causality.

 Activity 10.5

Review the sources of bias that you have considered in previous chapters

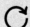 **Feedback**

Table 10.1 from the extract you considered in Chapter 2 summarises the main biases:

Table 10.1 Susceptibility of various designs to biases

| Design | Internal validity | | | | External validity | |
	Patient selection	Crossover	Error in measurement of outcomes	Error in ascertainment of exposure	Population	Technology
RCT	0	++	+	0	++	++
Non-RCT	+	+	+	0	+	+
CCS	++	0	+	+++	0	0
Comparison of clinical series	+++	0	+	0	+	+
Data bases	++	0	++	++	0	0

0 implies minimal vulnerability to a bias.
+++ implies high vulnerability to a bias.
RCT, randomized controlled trials; CCS, case-control studies.

Source: Eddy (1990)

Comparing study designs in action

Activity 10.6 gives you the opportunity to choose a study design to evaluate the effectiveness of a variety of interventions. Each of the examples could be evaluated using more than one design. However, certain study designs are more appropriate than others for particular situations. Each example is followed by a series of questions for which you will need to consider the main threats to the validity of the study designs that you propose. The feedback will suggest study designs for each intervention, together with some of the reasons why they are appropriate. Do not worry if you have chosen different study designs, so long as you are able to accurately justify your choice.

 Activity 10.6

This activity presents three examples of health interventions. Decide which study design is most appropriate for measuring the effectiveness of these interventions. You may find it useful to consider the following questions when choosing study designs:

1 Who is the study population?
2 Who is the wider population?
3 What is the intervention?
4 What is the outcome?
5 Which design will investigate the association between the intervention and outcome?
6 How would you analyse the results?
7 What measure of association would you use?
8 What threats to validity exist?

Example 1

A local council is worried because there has been a rise in road traffic accidents involving children. Many of these accidents have taken place on streets near a school. The council has been advised to introduce a number of traffic calming measures and a school crossing patrol (a person who stops the traffic to allow children to cross the street to reach the school). What study design would you use to evaluate the effectiveness of these measures in reducing road traffic accidents among children attending the school?

Feedback

Your answer should consider the following points:

1 *Who is the study population?* The study population could be defined as children who attend this particular school. Alternatively, it could be those children who live within a specified distance from the school.

2 *Who is the wider population?* Ideally, you would want to be able to generalize the results of this study to the wider population of all school-aged children.

3 *What is the intervention?* The intervention is the introduction of traffic calming measures and the school crossing patrol.

4 *What is the outcome?* The outcome to be measured is the rate of accidents in the children who make up the study population.

5 *Which design will investigate the association between the intervention and the outcome in this study population?* The intervention is applied to a population rather than to individuals. The traffic calming measures are an ecological exposure, and you cannot guarantee that the children will actually use the crossing patrol. It would therefore be reasonable to choose an ecological study design.

6 *How would you analyse the results?* You could use a single time-series study; that is, measuring the outcome before and after the intervention. This would mean measuring the annual rates of accidents in the study population over a number of years before the traffic calming measures. After these had been introduced, the annual accident rates would be measured again and the difference between rates before and after would be used as a measure of association between exposure and outcome. You could go further and use a multiple group design to compare the rates of accidents in schoolchildren from this study group with the rates in children attending schools without traffic calming measures or a school patrol.

7 *What measure of association would you use?* The measure of association would be determined by the method of analysis, but it could be a rate ratio or an odds ratio.

8 *What threats to validity exist?* Bias may occur because of changes in behaviour after the introduction of the new measures. For example, parents may actually be more likely to allow their children to walk to school unsupervised if they know that there is a crossing patrol. This could lead to a smaller decrease in accident rates than you would expect. In a multiple group design, the effect of any other initiatives (a concurrent intervention) to reduce accidents would need to be taken into account in any comparisons. The accident rate could also be confounded by seasonal variations.

 Example 2

The Ministry of Health would like to test a new vaccine, which has been developed to prevent malaria. The vaccine is expensive, but malaria causes an enormous burden of ill health in this country. The standard methods of controlling malaria rely on vector control (insecticides and drainage programmes). The pharmaceutical company that produces this vaccine will fund studies to measure its effectiveness. What study design would you use to evaluate the effectiveness of the vaccine?

 Feedback

Your answer should consider the following points:

1 *Who is the study population?* The study population could be defined those who live in areas where malaria is endemic.

2 *Who are the wider population?* Ideally you would want to be able to generalize the results of this study to the general population of the country and possibly beyond.

3 *What is the intervention?* Immunization of individuals with complete courses of the new vaccine.

4 *What is the outcome?* The outcome to be measured is the incidence of episodes of clinical malaria in the study population.

5 *Which design will investigate the association between the intervention and outcome in this study population?* This is a new intervention with unknown effectiveness. It is probably reasonable to use an RCT. Although the intervention is applied to individuals, immunization may produce herd immunity if a sufficient proportion of the population becomes immune and if mosquitoes do not bring parasites from other communities. This is an important part of the measure of effectiveness. Therefore, it would be reasonable to randomize groups of people – perhaps whole villages – to receive the vaccine or not. It would probably not be ethical to use a placebo vaccine, because of the pain and inconvenience without any benefit to the subjects.

6 *How would you analyse the results?* If you randomized individuals to receive vaccine or no vaccine, you could calculate the rates of clinical malaria in vaccinated and unvaccinated individuals and calculate the rate ratio, or the vaccine's effectiveness. However, randomizing individuals would not take any account of the herd immunity that would be gained if enough of the local population became immune to interrupt the cycle of transmission. If you randomized groups of people, such as entire villages, you could calculate the rates of clinical malaria in villages receiving the vaccination programme, and the rates in villages that did not receive the vaccinations. Then you could calculate the rate ratio. Any pre-existing differences in underlying rates of malaria before the RCT began would need to be taken into account.

7 *What measure of association would you use?* The measure of association would be represented by the risk ratio or rate ratio comparing numbers (or rates) of episodes of clinical malaria in vaccinated or unvaccinated villages.

8 *What threats to validity exist?* Randomization can remove selection bias only if there are enough subjects randomized. So the sample size matters. If you are randomizing villages, you need to have a large enough number of villages to ensure equal distribution of confounding variables. Confounding could occur through differences in the methods used to control mosquitoes. There could also be differences in the age or socio-economic structure of different villages. There might even be differences in the reporting or diagnosis of malaria. Individual randomization would reduce the effects of these confounding variables. Differences in reporting (a form of observation bias) could be tackled by having a standard set of diagnostic criteria for clinical malaria. If the investigator who determined which cases fulfilled these criteria did not know who received the vaccine, this would further reduce bias.

Example 3

There have been a number of reports of serious adverse events in patients receiving long-term treatment with drug X. This drug is an extremely effective analgesic that has proved effective in sufferers from severe arthritis. Because it is expensive, it has only been used with patients who could not benefit from other analgesics. These patients do not want to be denied further supplies of drug X. However, there have been a number of cases of sudden death in patients treated with this drug. What study design would you use to determine whether there is a real increase in sudden deaths among patients taking drug X?

↻ Feedback

1 *Who are the study population?* The study population could be defined as patients with a diagnosis of arthritis (perhaps a specific type of arthritis).

2 *Who are the wider population?* Any adverse events of drug X will be assumed to apply to the general population unless there is a special reason to believe that only arthritis patients would suffer these effects.

3 *What is the intervention?* Having a prescription for drug X (perhaps for a minimum period of time).

4 *What is the outcome?* The outcome is sudden death. This may be defined as unexpected death which does not follow a diagnosis of life-threatening illness. It may be difficult to obtain enough information from death certificates alone. You may have to investigate the deaths of a large number of arthritis sufferers in order to determine which would actually count as sudden deaths.

5 *Which design will investigate the association between the intervention and outcome?* A cohort study may be able to evaluate the association between drug X and sudden death. You would define the exposed cohort as being arthritis sufferers treated with drug X. The unexposed cohort would be arthritis sufferers who were not treated with drug X. The design could be either prospective or retrospective. A prospective cohort study might take a long time to obtain enough outcome events to show evidence of a statistical association. A retrospective cohort study might have trouble obtaining adequate follow-up information and accurate data on the intervention. If the outcome is rare (which is quite likely in the case of sudden death), a case-control design might be more efficient. You would define cases as arthritis sufferers who had experienced a sudden death. Controls could be arthritis sufferers who had not experienced a sudden death.

6 *How would you analyse the results?* For a cohort study, you would measure the incidence of sudden death in the cohort exposed to drug X and in the unexposed cohort. You would then calculate a risk ratio. Alternatively, you could measure rates and then calculate a rate ratio. For a case-control study, you would measure the odds of exposure to drug X in the cases and in the controls. You would then calculate an odds ratio.

7 *What measure of association would you use?* If you chose a cohort study, you would need to calculate a risk ratio or a rate ratio. If you chose a case-control study, you would have to calculate an odds ratio.

8 *What threats to validity exist?* The main sources of bias in a cohort study are observation bias, and losses to follow-up. Observation bias can be reduced if the observer is

blind to the exposure status of subjects. There might be confounding by severity of disease because drug X was reserved for those patients with arthritis who were resistant to other types of analgesia. This might be overcome by stratifying the analysis by a measure of severity of arthritis. Age and sex might also be confounding variables. The duration of treatment with drug X might affect the probability of sudden death. This could mean that patients treated with drug X for only one or two years might show little increase in mortality, whereas those treated for many years might show a large increase in mortality. This could be determined by analysing those treated with a longer duration of drug X separately from those treated with a shorter duration. The main sources of bias in a case-control study are selection bias and observation bias. To reduce selection bias, you might match cases and controls so that they suffered from the same type of arthritis. Similarly, you might match them so that they had suffered from arthritis for similar periods of time. If the patients receiving drug X (the cases) tended to be hospitalized, you would select controls from other hospitalized arthritis patients if possible. Observation bias might interfere with the way that exposure was ascertained. Details of treatment with drug X would have to be obtained from prescription records. Confounding would present much the same problem as for cohort studies. Age, sex, severity of arthritis and co-morbidities could all cause confounding. Their effect could be reduced by stratifying the analyses by age, sex and the other suspected confounders.

Quality of evidence for effectiveness

When evaluating effectiveness, some study designs have higher internal validity than others. Systematic reviews of RCTs are considered to have the highest internal validity. Systematic reviews of RCTs involve statistical meta-analysis to combine the results of relevant trials, including those that have never been published. The purpose of meta-analysis is to increase statistical power and resolve the uncertainty when trials disagree. This technique also helps to improve the estimation of the size of the effect and may answer questions not posed at the start of individual trials. A systematic review has particular advantages when definitive trials are impossible or impractical, results of trials are conflicting or results of definitive trials are awaited. The Cochrane Collaboration is an international initiative which supports scientists and clinicians in carrying out systematic reviews of specific topics. This network provides a comprehensive database, not only on RCTs but also on observational studies that have been conducted on a topic.

Summary

Often, more than one study design is appropriate to evaluate the effectiveness of a particular intervention. Designs differ in terms of cost, complexity and the time it will take for them to provide an answer. They also differ in the measures of association that they can provide. The RCT is generally regarded as the most internally valid method of assessing effectiveness, although its results may not be very generalizable. It can provide evidence with which to judge causality. The measure of association is the risk ratio or odds ratio. The cohort study is ideal for a rare intervention. It can show the temporal relationship between exposure and out-come. Confounding is the main threat to validity. The measure of association is the risk ratio or odds ratio. The case-control study is ideal for evaluating rare outcomes, particularly where the intervention is reasonably common. This design does not show the temporal relationship between exposure and outcome. Selection bias is the main threat to validity. The measure of association is the odds ratio. Ecological studies evaluate interventions, outcomes or both at the level of groups. They are ideal for measuring the effects of policy interventions. The ecological fallacy limits their ability to provide evidence of causality. Analysis can be complex. The measure of association may be the risk ratio or the odds ratio.

References

Ball C, Richardson SW, Rosenburg W and Haynes RB (1996) *Evidence based on call*. Edinburgh: Churchill Livingstone.

Eddy DM (1990) Should we change the rules for evaluating medical technologies? in Gelijins AC (ed.) *Modern methods of clinical investigation*. Washington, DC: National Academy Press.

SECTION 4

Measuring cost and evaluating cost-effectiveness

11 Measuring cost

Overview

In addition to being effective, a health care evaluation must also be good value for money. Where there is a choice of alternative interventions, it is prudent to choose those that provide the greatest health gain for the available resources. This is the justification for measuring cost-effectiveness as part of a health care evaluation. This chapter will review some key economic concepts and processes that are of particular relevance to health care evaluation. You will consider the types of cost that need to be taken into account, which people and institutions bear these costs and how costs can be estimated.

Learning objectives

By the end of this chapter you should be better able to:

- describe why cost is important in health care evaluation
- discuss the basic terminology used to describe costs (financial and economic costs, recurrent and capital costs, direct, indirect and intangible costs)
- describe how to identify the costs for all relevant parties in a health care intervention
- describe the stages of performing a cost analysis (identification, measurement, valuation)
- explain the concepts of time preference and discounting

Key terms

Capital cost The value of capital resources which have useful lives greater than one year.

Cost The value of resources usually expressed in monetary terms.

Direct costs Resources used in the design, implementation, receipt and continuation of a health care intervention.

Discount rate The rate at which future costs and outcomes are discounted to account for time preference.

Discounting A method for adjusting the value of costs and outcomes which occur in different time periods into a common time period, usually the present.

Financial (budgetary) costs The accounting cost of a good or service usually representing the original (historical) amount paid as distinct from the opportunity cost.

Fixed costs A cost of production that does not vary with the level of content.

Indirect costs The value of resources expended by patients and their carers to enable individuals to receive an intervention.

Intangible costs The costs of discomfort, pain, anxiety or inconvenience.

Opportunity (economic) cost The value of the next best alternative forgone as a result of the decision made.

Recurrent cost The value of recurrent resources with useful lives of less than one year that have to be purchased at least once a year.

Time preference People's preference for consumption (or use of resources) now rather than later because they value present consumption more than the same consumption in the future.

Variable cost A cost of production that varies directly with the level of output.

Why is cost information important?

The principal justification for including cost analysis in evaluation of health care is that resources are scarce. Whenever a cost is used for a particular intervention this means that these resources are not available elsewhere. This is what economists refer to as 'opportunity cost'. As there is always a choice about how to use resources (including doing nothing), using systematic methods to determine costs and benefits ensures that resources are allocated in the most appropriate way. This may involve comparisons between health interventions or between different providers. Comparison of the distribution of resources between different regions, countries or populations is an important tool is evaluating equity. This will be discussed in more detail in Chapters 16 and 17. A cost analysis can also be used to identify the money spent on an intervention and to give a proper account of its use. It is a useful tool for planning a service, particularly when considering whether it will be sustainable and for estimating the resources that could be liberated from terminating a service.

Financial versus economic costs

In estimating costs it is important to distinguish between financial and economic costs. Financial costs are the actual monetary expenditure for the resources. Determining the financial cost of an intervention would include a description of the expenditure on the intervention, measurement of the amounts of inputs purchased (i.e. those items that are actually bought, including material, labour and hire of equipment) and valuation of items in terms of their market price. Financial cost can be considered from the perspective of any individual or organization. It also involves identifying the funds actually needed to cover the costs and indicating whether the intervention is affordable (Phillips *et al.* 1993).

Economic (or opportunity) cost is the cost of losing some alternative that would have brought a benefit. Determining the economic cost would include a description of the value of the opportunities lost in employing resources on this intervention, measurement of all resources employed in the intervention, including voluntary labour and donated goods, and valuation of resources in terms of opportunity costs (where the prices of a commodity do not actually represent the opportunity cost, a shadow price may be estimated). Economic cost is also combined with measures of effectiveness to show whether an intervention is cost-effective (Phillips *et al.* 1993). Cost-effectiveness will be discussed in more detail in Chapter 12.

Inputs

Like any other process, a health care intervention can be considered to consume various resources or inputs in order to produce health outputs. In general, costs can be defined as the value of the resources that are used. However, there are a number of different types of cost. Costs are usually considered in terms of the inputs that are purchased. For example, you count all the resources that are put into a particular service or intervention and measure their costs. In these situations the costs can be described as *recurrent costs* if they represent ongoing operating costs or *capital costs* if they are costs of resources with a useful life of more than one year. Capital costs are usually annualized, which means the cost is spread over a number of years, though it may be modified to take account of depreciation. Considering costs in this way is relatively straightforward and can make use of accounting information alone. It also enables comparisons to be made between different interventions.

It is also helpful to consider costs as *direct, indirect* and *intangible* costs. Direct costs are the value of resources that are directly attributable to the intervention (e.g. in the design, implementation, receipt or continuation of the intervention) and that require a payment to someone. These can be subdivided into health care costs (such as the cost of the treatment or the medical staff) and non-health care costs, which are not exclusively resources from the health care sector (such as the cost of transport to and from health care facilities). Indirect costs are the value of resources expended to enable individuals to receive the intervention (e.g. time spent waiting and foregone earnings). Indirect costs are usually measured in terms of wages or earnings that are lost. If this information is not available, indirect costs can be measured in terms of time and the value of activities that would have been done by the person if he/she had not spent time receiving the intervention. Intangible costs are the value of discomfort, pain, anxiety or inconvenience. These costs are difficult to measure and are rarely included in economic evaluations.

Activity 11.1 will give you an opportunity to consider each of these types of cost in relation to a specific health intervention.

Activity 11.1

Imagine you have been asked to plan a vaccination programme for a small village, which is situated a long way from the nearest large town. You want to vaccinate all the children in the village. List all the costs that you can anticipate, including those borne by the health service and also those borne by the patients. For each cost identify who will have to bear the cost.

 Feedback

There are a number of ways to approach a problem of this sort. It is probably easiest to imagine first the process of buying the vaccine and transporting it from the supplier to the village. Then you can consider the process of administering the vaccine to the recipients. You should also consider the costs incurred by the recipients themselves and their families and by the institutions involved. Such an institution could be an external donor organization, or any agency that is financing this vaccination programme, such as government or a non-governmental organization (NGO).

Costs borne by institutions

1 The vaccine is purchased from a supplier = cost of vaccine.

2 The vaccine is transported from the supplier to the village = cost of refrigerator + vehicle hire + fuel + driver.

3 The vaccine is stored in the village = cost of renting space + cost of running refrigerator.

4 Vaccine is administered to villagers = cost of paying health care workers + cost of equipment for vaccinating villagers (various disposable items, such as needles, syringes, swabs, disinfectant).

5 Records must be maintained = cost of clerical worker + necessary stationery.

6 Various items require disposal = cost of suitable containers + removal to appropriate waste facility.

7 If the health care workers and clerical staff do not live in the village, there will be costs incurred in transporting them, feeding them and perhaps paying for their accommodation.

Costs borne by villagers

1 Time spent waiting for vaccination = wages lost or other work foregone.

2 Discomfort after vaccination = reduced ability of parents to work or perform other necessary tasks because of caring for children.

3 Travel costs = villagers may need to pay for travel to the place where the vaccination will occur.

4 Accommodation, etc. for health care workers (if they don't pay for this themselves).

5 Payment towards the cost of vaccination = whatever they are charged. Note that this may reduce the costs to the donor organization(s).

From the list above, it appears that all institutional costs are direct costs. Most of the costs borne by the children who receive the vaccine, and their parents, are indirect. However, it is not unusual for parents to be asked to pay part of the cost of health care for their children. From the list above, there are only a few intangible costs.

Sources of cost information

In order to ensure that costs are estimated accurately, it is important to use financial data that are appropriate for the purpose. Such information may be collected from many sources, and some are more useful and reliable than others.

Accounts versus budgets

It is relatively straightforward to use organizations' accounts to calculate the costs that have been incurred by a programme (assuming that adequate records have been kept). This should tell you accurately the amount that was spent. Inevitably, it does not allow for changes in the techniques that will be used in the future.

Accounts could tell you how much was spent vaccinating children in particular villages last year, but would give you no idea whether the task might have been performed more efficiently. For example, were more health care workers employed than was strictly necessary? It is possible that a new technique is now available that could do the same job more efficiently. Perhaps the use of a high-pressure injector gun could vaccinate children more quickly and avoid the need to hire overnight accommodation for the workers.

Budgets can allow for the technical changes and expected changes in the costs of labour and materials. However, their figures are forecasts of future spending and cannot accurately reflect the effect of unforeseen circumstances, such as failure of the refrigerator requiring the purchase of both a new refrigerator and new vaccine supplies.

Valuation

Whatever sources of information are used, it is essential that all costs are measured in the same financial units. This involves calculating all costs in the same currency (usually the local currency) and relating these to the same period of time. The value of donated goods or time should also be included.

Stages in performing a cost analysis

In order to ensure that costs are considered methodically, three discrete stages of cost analysis have been suggested: identification, measurement and valuation.

Stage 1: identification

Start by describing the health care intervention that will be considered in the analysis. If you plan to leave out any parts of the intervention from the cost analysis, you should explain why they are not included. Then there are five steps you will need to take:

1 Identify all contributors to the intervention.
2 Identify all levels at which the intervention runs – local, district, regional, national or international.
3 Specify the perspective to be taken – recipient of the intervention, institution, health sector, government, society etc.
4 Decide on the time period for the analysis. If the costs are fairly constant over a number of years, annual cost information may be sufficient.
5 Identify resources used according to a common system of classification, such as recurrent and capital costs.

Stage 2: measurement

Once all the costs have been identified, they must be measured in appropriate units, such as hours of work or ampoules of vaccine. Joint costs (i.e. costs for services/equipment that are used for more than one health intervention) must be allocated to specific interventions

Stage 3: valuation

Goods and services are usually valued in terms of local currency at current prices. The value of donated goods and services is estimated in the same units. Where the prices of goods and services do not actually reflect their true worth, adjustments must be made.

Assessing shared costs

Sometimes particular personnel and equipment are used for more than one health intervention. Health care staff rarely perform only one intervention and premises usually have several different uses. When considering the cost of one specific intervention, it is necessary to calculate the proportion of shared costs that can be allocated to this intervention. This is usually calculated by estimating the proportion of staff time that is spent on the specific intervention and applying this to the hourly cost of labour. The cost of premises (including heating and lighting) is often allocated on the proportion of space occupied by recipients of the specific intervention.

You should also think of overhead costs. These shared resources are a prerequisite to the functioning of any organization and include, for example, general administrative services, land and general maintenance. These costs are also usually allocated on the basis of staff time or space used.

Activity 11.2 will give you an opportunity to choose the appropriate units for measuring costs. You will also determine how much of each input can be allocated to one specific intervention.

Activity 11.2

Suppose you were costing an oral rehydration programme to treat children with diarrhoeal illnesses. Consider the following inputs:

- staff
- materials
- buildings
- vehicles
- equipment

1 What units could you use to measure each of these inputs?
2 Suppose that staff, buildings, vehicles and equipment are shared with other programmes. Materials are solely used for producing the oral rehydration service (ORS). How would you apportion these inputs to the ORS programme? How would you take account of overhead costs?
3 How would you value these inputs?

Answer questions 1 and 2 by completing Table 11.1. The first line has been filled in for you.

Table 11.1 Measuring inputs

Input	Units of measurement	Proportion of input used for ORS
Staff	Time	Percentage staff time spent on ORS
Materials or equipment for ORS Buildings* Vehicles*		

* Consider both capital and recurrent costs

 Feedback

Your completed table should look something like Table 11.2.

Table 11.2 Inputs measured

Input	Units of measurement	Proportion of input used for ORS
Staff	Time	Percentage staff time spent on ORS
Materials or equipment for ORS	Weight	All materials used for producing ORS
Buildings*	Space	Square metres used for producing ORS
Vehicles*	Distance or time	Total distance (or trips) used to collect material for ORS production

* Consider both capital and recurrent costs

3 All costs would be valued using current prices in local currency.

Discounting

When performing a cost-effectiveness analysis, it is important that the values of costs and benefits are related to the same period of time. In general, people prefer benefits now but costs later, whereas in health care it is often necessary to pay the cost now and receive the benefit at some point in the future. The concepts of time preference and discounting provide a means of accounting for this dilemma. The text below by Wonderling *et al.* (2005) explains the concepts of time preference and discounting in more detail.

📖 Time preference and discounting

Costs and outcomes often occur at different times. Many people place a different value on costs and outcomes that occur in the future compared with those which occur sooner. Other things being equal, you'd probably rather receive health outcomes (save money, and decrease morbidity and mortality) now and pay for the interventions later. Unfortunately, especially when it comes to preventing disease, the opposite is usually true. We often have to pay for the interventions now and receive the benefits later. The example of hepatitis B vaccine illustrates this – you have to pay for the vaccination now but receive the outcomes much later (fewer cases of hepatitis, chronic liver disease, and liver cancer).

In conducting economic evaluations, this observation presents a dilemma. Because people do not place equal value on costs or outcomes that occur this year and those that occur in later years, economic evaluation must also value these costs and outcomes differently. While there are theoretical and practical problems, many economic evaluations are performed using some sort of adjustment for the occurrence over time, or discounting, both for costs and for outcomes.

Discounting is a way to adjust future costs (and outcomes) to today's equivalent costs (and outcomes) – termed the present value. The discount rate is the rate at which future costs and outcomes are discounted to account for time preference. The discount rate used is usually between 3% and 5%, when zero inflation is assumed (a 'real' discount rate). In some countries, the central government imposes a specific real discount rate when economic evaluations are performed for publicly funded projects. In other countries where no specific rate is imposed, the economists frequently choose one rate and then perform sensitivity analysis to ensure the conclusions are stable with respect to the assumption about discount rates.

However, discounting is controversial. Drummond and colleagues (1997) give an example of a comparison of two ways to reduce deaths from heart disease. One is an expansion of funding for coronary artery bypass grafting (CABG) and the other is a health education campaign to influence diet and lifestyle which would not yield benefits for some time to come. So if time preference and discount rate are used, CABG will look more attractive than the preventive campaign.

Discounting is a concept not accepted by all economists. While the majority agree that time preference exists empirically, the theoretical foundation of time preference, especially as regards health, is not very well established. In terms of costs, most economists agree that future and present costs are interchangeable with the use of money interest rates which reflect the opportunity cost of using funds today rather than in the distant future. However, controversies surface when discounting is applied to outcomes because outcomes are not as interchangeable as money. For instance, do people really as a general rule place a lesser value on future *health* outcomes? This implies that we really care less about future generations.

Summary

The measurement of costs in heath care evaluation is primarily justified by the need to obtain maximum health gain from the available health resources. When planning an evaluation it is necessary to decide which costs are important and to identify all institutions and individuals who actually bear the cost. You also need to consider the perspective from which the evaluation is performed. This will influence the range of costs it is particularly important to include. The costs associated with an intervention are described as inputs and can be classified in a number of ways. Recurrent (operating) costs and capital costs are allocated to the intervention according to the proportion that each intervention consumes relative to other interventions. Costs can also be described as fixed or variable. Direct costs represent payments for items or services. Indirect costs represent loss of time or opportunities foregone. Intangible costs represent the cost associated with pain or distress. Financial costs represent expenditure on resources whereas economic costs are based on opportunity costs. They indicate whether an intervention represents an efficient use of resources.

A cost analysis determines the resources used by a health care intervention or programme and involves three main stages: identification of the relevant inputs measurement if the amount of each input used, valuation of each input. All costs should be measured in appropriate units and valued at the same point in time, by discounting if necessary. When determining the costs of an intervention, you should take account of shared resources, including overhead costs.

References

Drummond MF, O'Brien B, Stoddart GL and Torrance GW (1997) *Methods for the economic evaluation of health care programmes*, 2nd edn. Oxford: Oxford University Press.

Phillips M, Mills A and Dye C (1993) *Guidelines for cost-effectiveness analysis of vector control programmes*, WHO/CWS/93.4. Geneva: WHO.

Wonderling D, Gruen R, and Black N (2005) *Introduction to health economics*. Maidenhead: Open University Press.

12 Evaluating cost-effectiveness

Overview

In the previous chapter you reviewed the measurement and analysis of costs in health care. Economic evaluation involves a number of techniques, which combine measurement of cost with measurement of outcomes. This makes it possible to compare interventions in order to obtain the maximum health gain for a given expenditure, or the lowest expenditure for a given health gain. This chapter will focus on cost-effectiveness and cost-utility analysis as the principle designs that are relevant to health care evaluation.

Learning objectives

Bt the end of the chapter the student should be better able to:

* **outline the basic principals of economic analysis**
* **describe the steps necessary to perform a cost-effectiveness analysis**
* **critically evaluate cost-effectiveness and cost-utility analysis**

Key terms

Cost-benefit analysis An economic evaluation technique in which outcomes are expressed in monetary terms.

Cost-effectiveness analysis Economic evaluations with outcomes measured in health units.

Cost minimization A method of economic analysis for comparing the costs of different interventions which produce the same outcome.

Cost-utility analysis Economic evaluations where the outcomes are measured in health units which capture not just the quantitative but also the qualitative aspects of the outome, such as quality of life.

Economic analysis A general term for a number of related techniques which seek to identify, measure, value and compare the costs and consequences of alternative actions.

Quality-adjusted life years (QALYs) A numerical representation of the value attached to a combination of quantity and quality of life, where one year of perfect health is set at "1".

Utility values Numerical representation of the degree of satisfaction with health status, health outcome or health care.

Economic analysis

Economic analysis is a general term for a number of related techniques which seek to identify, measure, value and compare the costs and consequences of alternative actions (Drummond *et al.* 1987). They can be used to help choose between alternative health care interventions in order to maximize the health gain for a given use of resources. Such analyses can also help to determine health care priorities. It is important to realize that the issues being addressed are of considerable public importance, as providing treatment for some individuals may involve denying treatment to others.

Types of economic analysis

There are a number of different techniques that can be used to compare the costs and outputs of two or more health care interventions. Activity 12.1 will enable you to describe the most important ones.

 Activity 12.1

Read the extract below by Watson (1997) that describes the main methods of economic evaluation. As you read this passage, consider the relative usefulness of each of the following in health care evaluation:

1 Cost minimization analysis.
2 Cost-effectiveness analysis.
3 Cost-benefit analysis.
4 Cost-utility analysis.

 Cost-minimization analysis

Cost-minimization analysis can be used to evaluate the costs of alternative therapies which generate exactly the same clinical outcomes. This approach therefore evaluates on the basis of technical efficiency. Clinical effectiveness would be established by randomized control trial, and then the choice between alternative interventions would be determined according to whichever treatment was cheapest. Various studies comparing in-patient treatment of minor conditions requiring surgery with out-patient treatment have been conducted using this approach.

Cost-effectiveness analysis

If the clinical outcomes of alternative therapies differ, then the consequences as well as the costs of each procedure need to be considered as part of their economic evaluation. If the effectiveness of the alternative procedures can be expressed in terms of a common unit of measurement such as life years saved or pain-free days gained, then they can be evaluated on the basis of cost-effectiveness, i.e. for each procedure, cost per pain-free day, or cost per life year gained, could be compared . . . Cost-effectiveness analysis is limited by the need to express outcomes in the same units. If this is not possible, because outcomes have more than one dimension, then some more sophisticated evaluation of the benefits derived from a procedure is required.

Cost-benefit analysis

Cost-benefit analysis seeks to place a money valuation on both the costs and benefits of alternative treatments in order to determine the net benefit (i.e. benefits minus costs) accruing from each programme. One advantage with this approach is that it also facilitates comparison between the net benefits gained from a given level of expenditure on health care and those which would follow from the same sum being spent on alternative services, such as education or transport. This method of analysis could therefore be helpful in determining the optimal proportion of GDP [gross domestic product] to allocate to the health care.

The difficulty of cost-benefit analysis of health care is how to value the benefits accurately. Two approaches have generally been adopted. The first method is derived from human capital theory. This treats health care as an investment in human capital which will yield a return once the individual recovers and returns to work. That return could be valued as a discounted stream of future income. Unfortunately, this approach is incomplete since it values benefits by reference to productive potential valued at the market rate for that individual. This makes unrealistic assumptions about the labour market being competitive, and omits a personal appraisal of benefits, both direct and indirect. This approach, then, measures benefit in terms of livelihoods rather than lives. This would imply, for example, that the benefits from treating a highly paid professional would exceed those gained by treating a low paid worker, even if their conditions and post-operative prognoses were identical. It also creates obvious problems in valuing the benefits from treating people who have retired or who are unemployed.

An alternative approach is to value health care interventions by identifying how much people would be willing to pay to secure the benefits from a given treatment or to escape the costs of the related illness. However, this method also has its weaknesses. An individual's valuation of a treatment may be influenced by the framing of questions designed to elicit that valuation. Individuals have also been shown to vary their valuations according to whether they suffer from the illness concerned, and according to their income. These problems may become more acute the more severe the condition under consideration or the larger the valuation attached to treatment.

Given this range of responses, the sample of individuals surveyed in the willingness to pay surveys from which benefit valuations are derived should either be identified using stratified random sampling techniques to reflect differences in income and health status, or their responses should be weighted to reflect these characteristics in the population. If the latter option is taken, a further problem is then how to select the appropriate weights for these responses.

Cost-utility analysis

Rather than trying to express benefits as a monetary valuation, benefits could be valued in terms of utility. Utility refers to a subjective assessment of the well-being gained from alternative interventions. This measure therefore takes account of qualitative as well as quantitative medical outcomes.

The most common approach is to adjust the number of life years gained from an intervention by the quality of life enjoyed by those treated. This method allows a more sophisticated appreciation of cost-effectiveness. If, for example, a condition can be treated in two ways which produce different outcomes in terms of mortality and say, subsequent patient mobility, simple cost-effectiveness would be an inappropriate method of economic evaluation to adopt since it could not capture both dimensions, mortality and mobility. If, however, the full implications of impaired mobility could be rated using a quality of life index, these two features of medical outcome could be combined into a single measurement of the benefits from treatment. This would enable evaluation of alternative programmes to be made on the basis of cost per quality-adjusted life year (QALY).

The challenge with this approach is how to assess the multifarious factors which constitute the quality of life. Various clinical profiles have been developed to try to assess qualitative medical outcomes. These include, for example, the Functional Limitations Profile, the Nottingham Health Profile (NHP), and the SF-36 . . . These assess health status on a range of dimensions such as social interaction, pain, emotional functioning, mobility, etc. However, one of the limitations of multi-dimensional assessments is that comparison of outcomes between different conditions is difficult since different dimensions within the profile may assume varying degrees of significance according to the disease under consideration. While these profiles permit comparison of health status for alternative treatments of the same condition, economic evaluation to determine resource allocation between conditions would be impossible (or, at best, imprecise). In order for economic analysis to be meaningful the quality of life needs to be expressed as a single index which could then be combined with measures of mortality to identify a QALY.

In order to generate a single unit index of life quality three issues must be addressed. First, the relevant dimensions of life quality need to be determined. Second, utility must be measured for each dimension. Finally, valuations of utility for each dimension need to be aggregated.

↻ Feedback

1 Cost minimization analysis can be used to compare the costs of any interventions that treat the same illness and have the same clinical outcomes – two different surgical techniques which have identical clinical results, for instance. If the outcomes are the same, you simply choose the cheapest intervention.

2 Cost-effectiveness analysis can be used to compare interventions so long as they produce health outcomes that can be measured using the same units. For example, you could compare interventions which measured their outcomes in terms of the cost per life year gained. Cost-effectiveness analysis tends to focus on a single measure of health outcome that is common to all the interventions being compared. Cost-effectiveness studies are most frequently used in health care evaluation and they are relatively easy to perform. Cost minimization is just a special case of a cost-effectiveness study where the outcomes produced by the interventions are the same.

3 Cost-benefit analysis involves calculating a monetary value for both the costs and consequences of the intervention. It can compare any interventions that produce outcomes which can be measured in financial terms.

4 Cost-utility analysis involves expressing the health outcomes in terms of utility (that is, quality-adjusted outcomes). It should be possible to compare any interventions using a cost-utility analysis, so long as their outcomes can be represented in terms of utilities.

However, it can be difficult to incorporate the different subjective factors that determine QoL into a single measure such as the QALY.

You should keep in mind that most often health care evaluation involves comparing two interventions that seek to address the same health need. This form of comparison is achieved by cost-effectiveness analysis, and this is the technique that will be described in more detail in the following section.

Steps in performing a cost-effectiveness analysis (CEA)

1 State the question to be evaluated. Identify the alternative interventions you want to compare. This may include the option to do nothing, which would represent the existing state before introducing a new form of health care. State the viewpoint from which the analysis is to be made.

2 Give a detailed description of the alternative interventions. It may help to consider them in terms of provider, process, recipient and frequency. These can be summarized as 'who' does 'what' to 'whom' 'where' and 'how often'.

3 Describe the outcome measures you are going to use, such as disease, health status, QoL measures. Identify the single common outcome measure that you want to use in comparing the interventions. This is usually the primary health outcome of the intervention.

4 Identify, measure and value all relevant costs and adjust if necessary for differential timing (discounting).

5 Now integrate costs with outcomes and calculate the cost-effectiveness ratio for each intervention. Determine the amount of outcomes improved per dollar spent – for example. $x/unit of outcomes (e.g. $5000/life year saved). Alternatively, you could calculate the amount of money needed to improve one unit of outcome. Compare the ratios of the different interventions and calculate the difference between the ratios to identify the cost-effective one. If outcomes are the same, choose the one with the lowest costs (cost minimization technique).

6 Perform a sensitivity analysis. Make reasonable assumptions on changes of key parameters that could affect the cost-effectiveness of the intervention. Sensitivity analysis is useful when there is uncertainty in the measurement of costs or outcomes; that is, where it is difficult to measure costs accurately or where a number of providers show very different performance for the same intervention. You could, for example, calculate the effect of price changes of one or more key inputs on the cost-effectiveness of the intervention. Or you could analyse how sensitive the cost-effectiveness ratio is to variations in performance. Alternatively, inputs can be changed to represent extreme situations – in the immunization example above, for example, you could estimate the effect of a tenfold rise in vaccine prices on the total cost of the programme.

7 In your results and discussion, present all relevant assumptions and their likely effects. Also, show how your calculated results may apply to other settings and discuss the extent to which they are generalizable.

Limitations of CEA

Though CEA is a useful tool in decision-making, it has some limitations:

1 Where two interventions are applied to different populations, the cost-effectiveness ratios may be confounded by differences in the populations.
2 A full CEA can be expensive and time-consuming.
3 It may be difficult to choose a single outcome indicator.
4 A CEA is of limited generalizability when key parameters change rapidly.

Combining quality and quantity

Cost-utility analysis is a method that compares interventions that value their outcomes in terms of a preference-based composite measure of health. Some health indices can be combined with the quantity of a person's remaining life to create an outcome measure, such as a QALY. To obtain this measure, people are asked to decide how much they value different states of QoL. QALYs have been used by the WHO to compare the outcomes of health care interventions in different populations and across very different clinical conditions. A similar approach can be taken using patients' values of different levels of disability or functional health status. When such measurements of function are applied to the estimated duration of life in a given state of health, you have a measure such as the disability-adjusted life year (DALY). This was developed by the World Bank to allow comparison between the outcomes of different interventions.

There are three main techniques for eliciting preferences. The most simple method is known as *magnitude estimation* and uses a rating scale such as a visual analogue scale where the top and bottom points are labelled. For example, the top of the scale is defined as the most desirable health state (perfect health) and the bottom is defined as the worst. The respondent is presented with a series of health state scenarios and is asked to imagine that they have lived in each state for a specified period of time, without change and with the same outcome at the end. The respondent then ranks each health state according to his or her preference and places them on the rating scale.

An alternative method of eliciting preferences is to use the time trade-off technique. This requires the respondent to choose between living in state A for x amount of time and living in state B for y amount of time where both states have the same final outcome. Time x and y are systematically varied until the respondent cannot choose between the two states. If time x is varied to find the point of indifference the time trade-off score for health state B is x/y.

The third method of eliciting preferences is more complex and includes health states that involve uncertainties. The respondent has to choose between two health states. Choice A is uncertain and has two possible outcomes. Choice B is a certain choice and has only one possible outcome. Both choices last for the same amount of time and are usually presented so that they are age-specific in terms of life expectancy. The probability of choice A is varied until the respondent is indifferent between the uncertain choice A and the certain choice B. The probability at the point of indifference is the utility of the health state in choice B.

There are a number of methodological difficulties in using these three methods. Firstly, the tasks, particularly time trade-off and standard gamble, are quite complex. It is not clear whether people understand clearly what is expected of them and/or whether they are able to do the task reliably. Secondly, the tasks involve hypothetical health states. It is possible that people give different preferences in relation to a hypothetical situation compared with a real health situation. Thirdly, the degree of risk aversion may differ between respondents. It is therefore difficult to distinguish whether differences in valuations reflect the condition or the characteristics of the individual.

✎ Activity 12.2

Read the following extract by Watson (1997). What are the advantages and disadvantages of using QALYs in the context of health care provision?

📖 Quality adjusted life years (QALYs)

QALYs are used as a single-index measure of health benefits which can then be applied in cost-effectiveness analysis. Life expectancy estimates (the quantity of life gained by intervention) are weighted by a quality of life quotient. If it is assumed that both quantity and quality of life are relevant parameters for health care appraisal, and these can be captured effectively in health related quality of life indicators, QALYs provide a useful source of information for health care managers seeking to evaluate the efficiency of alternative treatments, and also to prioritize the claim of competing health care projects on scarce resources.

The first problem to be addressed is . . . how to describe and value health-related quality of life. As we have seen, the various measures adopted in cost-utility analysis differ in their dimensions and/or in the valuation methodology. A further issue is to consider whose views should be taken into account in determining the quality of life associated with a condition. Again, empirical studies have varied according to whether a generic index (such as the Rosser index) is applied, or whether specific valuations are gained from patients suffering from the relevant condition, the general public, or from doctors.

Having established the relevant measure of quality of life, these quotients can then be applied to mortality data to determine the benefits from treatment expressed in terms of quality adjusted life years. Thus if the health-related quality of life score for a given condition is 0.8, one year of life in this state would be equivalent to 0.8 QALYs. Similarly, five years of life in a health state which achieved a quality of life score of just 0.5 would be equivalent to 2.5 QALYs. Since an intervention will not necessarily be successful, the QALYs associated with a successful procedure need to be moderated by the probability of success being achieved. If costs were then attached to each intervention, league tables of costs per QALY could be estimated for a range of procedures in order to facilitate economic evaluation.

This process can be illustrated if we consider an example of 100 patients who are the same age and suffer from the same condition (the first part of the example below follows the form outlined by Kind and Gudex 1993). Their initial health status is valued at 0.6 and they have a life expectancy of 20 years. Their condition can either be treated by surgery or by chemotherapy. Surgery has a probability of achieving a complete cure of 90 per cent, but a probability of death of 10 per cent; all the patients receiving chemotherapy survive, but their quality of life is only enhanced to 0.8. Which treatment is the most effective? If 50 patients are treated using each method, the two procedures can be compared as follows:

Surgery

Successful: QALYs are measured as the net gain in QALYs achieved by survivors over and above what they would have enjoyed had they not been treated, i.e.:

QALYs = (20 years × I) – (20 years × 0.6)

= 20 – 12 = 8 QALYs per patient

If 90 per cent of patients survive the operation then the total QALYs gained from successful surgery can be identified as:

0.9 (50) × 8 = 360 QALYs

Unsuccessful: QALYs are measured as the net loss *of* QALYs suffered by casualties of surgery below what they would have enjoyed had they never been treated, i.e.:

QALYs = 0 – (20 years × 0.6)

= – 12 QALYs per casualty

If 10 per cent of patients die during the operation, the net loss of QALYs can be identified as:

0.1 (50) × – 12 = –60 QALYs

So, the net effect of surgery on the 50 patients treated in this way is:

360 – 60 = 300 QALYs

= 6 QALYs per patient undergoing surgery.

Chemotherapy

QALYs here are found by the same method:

= (20 × 0.8) – (20 × 0.6)

= 16 – 12 = 4 QALYs per patient

= 200 QALYs for all 50 patients treated in this way

Thus the net benefit of receiving surgery rather than chemotherapy can be found by subtracting the total QALYs achieved by the latter treatment from the former, i.e. 100 QALYs.

If we wanted to determine which procedure was the most cost-effective, we could work out the relative costs per QALY. If an operation costs £1000, and drug treatment costs £25 per year for 20 years (i.e. £500 per patient), then the cost per QALY can be estimated for surgery at £166.67 and for drug treatment at £125. On this basis, chemotherapy would be shown to be more cost-effective.

Although QALYs have considerable potential for aiding decisions concerning health resource allocation, they have been subject to significant criticism. First, it has been argued that there are technical limitations in the quality of life indicators from which QALYs have been calculated. The original Rosser index is based on just 70 respondents from six categories, so there is a high probability of small sample error. However, this criticism is not valid for the EuroQol as valuations have been gained from much larger samples, with the largest sample to date being 3000. The test-retest reliability of these measures is often limited, and the various methodologies adopted to value utilities produce different results (Williams and Kind 1992). Some subjects have displayed difficulty in reporting consistent results using the standard gamble or time trade-off approaches to valuing utilities. Individual perceptions of risk may also differ, so some may prefer less time in a certain but poorer condition, whereas others would take the risk to achieve a higher health state. In addition, if subjects are drawn from different groups, such as patients, doctors and the healthy public, valuations range quite widely (Slevin *et al.* 1988). This problem could apply with respect to age, gender, ethnic origin and economic status, as well as according to health status. Furthermore, the basic principle of QALYs is that there is a constant proportional trade-off between length of life and health status, so ten years in a health state valued at 0.8 is assumed to be equivalent to eight years of perfect health and five years in the same health state would be equivalent to four years of perfect health. However, there may be a threshold effect where patients are only willing to trade length of life for greater quality once they are guaranteed a certain amount of future life. Certainly it is unlikely that the rate of trade-off will remain constant whatever the duration of life (Loomes and McKenzie 1989).

Other concerns focus on the use of QALYs in league tables. One problem may be that the cost per OALY is subject to how much money has already been invested into a programme. Cost per QALY may vary over time for a number of reasons. First, there may be economies of scale and experience as a new technique becomes adopted more widely resulting in lower costs per QALY. Second, if the patients who are treated first are those for whom the number of QALYs gained are highest per unit of costs, then as more is spent, patients must increasingly be being treated who yield fewer QALYs per unit of expenditure. Both of these influences suggest that league tables would have to be updated at regular intervals if they were to be an effective indicator of relative costs and benefits (Mooney 1994).

Ethical objections have also been levelled at QALYs focusing in particular on their implications for distributive justice and the equality principle. For example, although Harris accepts their contribution in evaluating alternative treatments for the same patient, he suggests that they are completely inappropriate for interpersonal comparison. QALYs are unjust because they do not allow equal access to resources according to need, they distribute according to the benefits gained per unit of cost. Harris maintains that this permits discrimination. He argues, for example, that ageism is an inevitable consequence of the adoption of QALYs, since other things being equal the elderly have a lower life expectancy than the young (Harris 1987). One defence of QALYs against the challenge of ageism (which Harris acknowledges) is that they prefer those with longer rather than shorter life expectancies, irrespective of age. Indeed it has been argued that QALYs are not ageist enough: if it is accepted that the elderly are fortunate to the extent that they have enjoyed a 'good innings' then justice considerations might advocate treating younger patients, even if they had lower life expectancies (Lockwood 1988). Indeed this view seems to be embraced by some health economists who claim that if we wish to equalize lifetime experience of health then those who have had a 'fair innings' should not expect to have as much spent on health improvement as younger people who seem less likely to lead such a healthy life (Williams 1997).

Justice conditions might also be violated by the case of people who suffer from rare conditions which [are] expensive to treat who would also be disadvantaged by QALYs. This could also create a problem of inefficiency since experimental treatments could be ruled out initially by their relative expense, even if as they were used more widely their cost would fall (Harris 1988). Economists might respond to this challenge by advocating a cost structure which discounts expenditure on research and development and compensates for uncertainties in the success of new treatment methods.

If health-related quality of life is considered to be an important factor to include in economic evaluations of health care, this raises a question as to why (other than for practical reasons) we should fail to take account of other qualitative factors in distributing health resources. QALYs allow treatment to be distributed to those who enjoy better rather than inferior health states, since the QALYs gained by intervention will be greater, other things being equal, in the former case. However QALYs do not advocate distribution on the basis of incomes, even if the quality of life of the rich were regarded as superior to that of the poor. Broome argues that this latter case is no more unfair than the former (Broome 1988).

Feedback

Advantages to using QALYs:

1 A single index that represents the quality, quantity and valuation of life is needed for cost-utility analyses.

2 The QALY can be used to compare the outcomes of different interventions applied to different diseases and different populations.

3 A common unit of analysis such as the QALY can help the process of explicit decision-making, particularly with regard to prioritization and resource allocation.

Disadvantages to using QALYs:

1 The ranking of states of health relies on hypothetical judgements. People may value health states differently when they are hypothetical compared with how they would value them if they actually experienced them.

2 Preferences and judgements are affected by the health and culture of the respondent. There is therefore an issue about which population is appropriate for eliciting preferences.

3 It is not always clear whose judgements should be considered (e.g. patients, doctors, the general public).

4 QALYs do not always provide a sufficiently sensitive measure for making clinical judgements.

5 There are methodological difficulties in obtaining preferences. Different elicitation techniques give different values for the same health state.

6 Ethical objections have been raised about the use of QALYs. Such measures mean that resource allocation decisions are less likely to favour the elderly as they have fewer years of life left in which to benefit. Similarly, QALYs can be used to justify a failure to treat small numbers of patients with rare, expensive conditions.

Summary

Economic analysis seeks to identify, measure, value and compare the costs and consequences of alternative actions. There are two main techniques of economic analysis that are applicable to health care evaluation – namely, cost-effectiveness analysis and cost-utility analysis.

References

Broome J (1988) Good, fairness and QALYs, in Bell M and Mendus S (eds) *Philosophy and medical welfare*. Cambridge: Cambridge University Press.

Drummond MF, O'Brien B, Stoddart GL and Torrance GW (1987) Cost analysis, in Drummond MF *et al. Methods for the economic evaluation of health care programmes*, 2nd edn. Oxford: Oxford University Press.

Harris J (1987) QALYfying the value of life. *Journal of Medical Ethics* 13: 117–23.

Harris J (1988) More and better justice, in Bell M and Mendus S (eds) *Philosophy and medical welfare*. Cambridge: Cambridge University Press.

Kind P and Gudex C (1993) The role of QALYs in assessing priorities between health care interventions, in Drummond MF and Maynard A (eds) *Purchasing and providing cost-effective health care*. London: Longman.

Lockwood M (1988) Quality of life and resource allocation, in Bell M and Mendus S (eds) *Philosophy and medical welfare*. Cambridge: Cambridge University Press.

Loomes G and McKenzie L (1989) The use of QALYs in health care decision making. *Social Science and Medicine* 28: 299–308.

Mooney G (1994) *Key issues in health economics*. London: Harvester Wheatsheaf.

Slevin ML, Plant H, Lynch D, Drinkwater J and Gregory WM (1988) Who should measure quality of life, the doctor or the patient? *British Journal of Cancer* 57: 109–12.

Watson K (1997) Economic evaluation of health care, in Jenkinson C (ed.) *Assessment and evaluation of health and medical care*. Buckingham: Open University Press.

Williams A (1997) Intergenerational equity: an exploration of the 'fair innings' argument. *Health Economics* 6: 117–32.

Williams A and Kind P (1992) The present state if play about QALYs, in Hopkins A (ed.) *Measures of the quality of life and the uses to which such measures may be put*. London: Royal College of Physicians of London.

SECTION 5

Evaluating humanity

Evaluating humanity

Overview

Financial restrictions mean that health care is often dominated by the need for efficiency. It is possible to consider health care as a number of production processes and forget the human beings who receive and provide care. Therefore, when evaluating health care, it is especially important to consider humanity as well as effectiveness and efficiency. This chapter will introduce the concept of humanity and some of the threats to it. It will also begin to consider how humanity might be evaluated in the context of health care evaluation.

Learning objectives

By the end of this chapter you should be better able to:

- **explain the various aspects of humanity and the relationship between concepts of humanity and patient satisfaction**
- **identify circumstances when health care could lack humanity**
- **outline how humanity might be evaluated in the context of health care**

Key terms

Autonomy The principle that human beings have free will and the right to make choices about their actions and about what happens to them.

Beneficence The principle of striving to do good.

Dignity The principle that human beings are worthy of respect and have the right to be treated with courtesy and with consideration for their feelings.

Non-maleficence The principle of avoiding harm.

The dimensions of humanity

Exploring humanity in health care evaluation means assessing the social, psychological and ethical acceptability of the way that people are treated by health services. The term 'humanity' describes the quality of being civil, courteous or obliging towards other people. It is characterized by sympathy with and consideration for others. A humane doctor or nurse does not inflict unnecessary discomfort on patients or relatives. Humanity also involves respect for the dignity and autonomy of patients and a commitment to maximize the benefits obtained by health care while minimizing any harm. In general, assessing humanity involves a range of activities in both management and research. These might include handling complaints, monitoring standards of care, investigating claims of inhumanity, assessing the impact of new technologies, and changes in service delivery. This chapter and Chapters 14 and 15 will focus on the last of these aspects and on the scientific approaches to evaluating humanity.

Inhumanity in health care often comes to public attention through media coverage of specific incidents, such as carelessness or negligence which has resulted in undue suffering or even death. There are four dimensions that make up humanity in the context of health care. These are: autonomy, dignity, beneficence and non-maleficence. These are rights that every patient (or recipient of health care) should be entitled to expect.

Autonomy represents the principle that human beings have free will and the right to make choices about their actions and about what happens to them. Considering health care, autonomy suggests that patients should have the right to refuse treatment and to be fully involved in decisions about their care.

Dignity represents the principle that human beings are worthy of respect and have the right to be treated with courtesy and with consideration for their feelings. In order to respect the concept of human dignity, it is necessary to accept that all human beings are equal. Without a commitment to equal treatment, there will always be some individuals whose dignity is valued less than others.

Beneficence represents the principle of striving to do good. This is the justification for any form of health care. There is no point in providing health care for someone unless you hope to improve their state of health. Where there is a choice of interventions, it is usual to provide the intervention which is likely to give the largest benefits.

Non-maleficence represents the principle of avoiding harm and you would certainly never intentionally inflict harm on patients. When delivering health care, it is usual to consider what effect the care will have on the individual receiving it. For example, you would not give patients medication to which they are known to be allergic. Where there is a choice of intervention, it is usual to provide the intervention with the fewest harmful side-effects.

Beneficence and non-maleficence are usually considered together, because they represent very similar things: the desire to do good and the desire to prevent harm. Both are respected when you seek to provide the health care with the most benefits and the fewest adverse events.

Ways of assessing humanity

Humanity in health care is often not considered except in its absence. Activity 13.1 is intended to help you think about the concept of humanity by considering how examples of inhumanity become noticed.

Activity 13.1

Think of a recent incident of inhumanity in health services that has been covered in the media. Describe briefly how it came to public attention. What other sources could you use to obtain information on inhumanity in health care?

Feedback

Media coverage of inhumane situations or events is the most common way of bringing inhumanity to public attention. This can be triggered, for example, by patient complaints, insider reports, reports from pressure groups or 'whistle-blowers'. Other sources of information include:

- the internal complaints system of a health care organization
- special reports or inquiries
- specific research (using either quantitative or qualitative methods)

For example, an independent inquiry in the UK was established into the death of David 'Rocky' Bennett, a black patient with schizophrenia who died after a struggle with nursing staff at a medium secure unit (Kmietowicz 2005). The report noted that the cultural needs of black and ethnic minorities are not yet adequately addressed and recommended an action plan to reduce the inequalities experienced by such patients in mental health services.

How can health care lack humanity?

It is easy to imagine how health care can be delivered in an inhumane way. Consider a psychiatric ward where patients are permanently restrained, or where they are not given enough food. Gross inhumanity should be rare in most systems of health care, however there are less obvious forms of inhumanity, inflicted by organizational needs, routine work and lack of consideration. Activity 13.2 is intended to give you the opportunity to think about ways in which health care provision may be less humane than it should be.

Activity 13.2

Write down some ways in which care may not be provided humanely in a hospital or health centre. Try to think of examples where carers may not realize that their practices are lacking in humanity.

Feedback

There are no right or wrong answers. Any lack of respect for individuals' dignity or autonomy would be inhumane. Humanity seeks to maximize benefits and minimize harm. If this is not achieved, you have a degree of inhumanity. Here are some examples of failures of humanity in a hospital:

Lack of respect for dignity
- refusal to permit patients to wear their own night-clothes
- isolating patients with human immunodeficiency virus (HIV) and making them wait for treatment in a separate area
- early waking times on hospital wards
- Friday afternoon discharge from hospital

Lack of respect for autonomy
- standing around patients' beds and discussing them as though they were not present
- not providing enough information about daily routines or what to expect
- vaccinating people without giving them a chance to make an informed choice as to whether they actually want the vaccination

Lack of commitment to beneficence
- providing the standard treatment when there is another treatment available that would be better for a specific individual

Lack of commitment to non-maleficence
- performing unnecessary and painful tests
- administering a drug to which the patient is known to be allergic

Limits to humanity

Achieving humanity is sometimes in conflict with other aims of health care. For example, there may be a conflict between the rights of the individual to expect humane health care and the behaviour of individual patients, the need for efficiency, or the needs of the community or society.

Just as we accept that patients have rights which define humane treatment, so we also have expectations of patients which might conflict with these rights. We expect patients to attend their appointments, answer questions truthfully (even very intimate questions) and comply with their treatment regimens. Under resource constraints there is pressure to run services efficiently to maximize health gain for the largest number of people. The need for increased throughput limits the time available for individual care and may jeopardize the quality of care. There may, thus, be a trade-off between efficiency and humanity. The immunization of children involves persuading parents to allow their children to be treated. Any serious adverse events which may be expected to happen to a very small minority are considered acceptable when compared to the reduction of illness in a whole population. However, they do not appear acceptable to the families whose children suffer these events. There are also limitations to humanity which are imposed by society. General views and attitudes prevailing in society may be reflected in health services. These preferences may lead to implicit rationing of resources and the provision of less humane services for disadvantaged groups such as the elderly, disabled and mentally ill.

How would you assess humanity in health care?

It is reasonable to assume that patients who are treated humanely are more likely to be satisfied with the health care processes that they have received than those whose treatment has been less humane. Notice that we are considering satisfaction with the way that health care is provided, not with the outcomes that are achieved. For the purposes of health care evaluation, measuring humanity will be taken to mean measuring satisfaction with the processes of care as they affect autonomy, dignity and beneficence (including non-maleficence). This involves assessing patients' experience of health care, including the behaviour of staff, the health care environment and the way in which patients are informed and empowered to participate in planning and managing their own treatment.

Detecting inhumanity

Inhumane treatment may lead to complaints. These can be valuable for detecting deficiencies in the provision of health care, but may not give a valid measure of the experience of most patients. Those who complain may not be typical of the majority. However, a lack of complaints does not mean that the service is satisfactory. There are large differences between countries as to the views held on the appropriateness of complaints and the cultural and legal conditions that promote patients' rights. For example, the frequency of complaints and litigation suits is much higher in the USA than in the UK, where the national culture is less supportive of complaining. Therefore, it may be necessary to assess humanity by more active means such as special visits, enquiries and surveys.

What affects patient satisfaction?

The next extract will demonstrate some of the aspects of health care that influence patient satisfaction.

 Activity 13.3

Read the extract below by Fitzpatrick (1997) about patient satisfaction. This passage mentions five areas of the health care experience which have a major effect on the amount of satisfaction expressed by patients. These five areas are: interpersonal skills (of health professionals); information giving (from health professionals); technical competence; the organization of health care; and time. Which of the dimensions of humanity (autonomy, dignity, beneficence and non-maleficence) would be assessed by measuring patient satisfaction in each of these five areas?

 What is patient satisfaction?

... detailed research has shown that patients are capable of making quite complex and differentiated judgements of the quality of their care so that the construct is most usefully considered as multi-dimensional (Table 13.1). Thus patients may hold distinct and

Table 13.1 Dimensions of patient satisfaction

• Humaneness	• Cost
• Informativeness	• Facilities
• Overall quality	• Outcome
• Competence	• Continuity
• Bureaucracy	• Attention to psychosocial problems
• Access	

Source: Fitzpatrick (1997)

independent views on the one hand as to whether the health professionals from whom they have received care are humane and have good interpersonal skills, and on the other hand regarding the costs or accessibility of services ... How investigators define patient satisfaction and which aspects they choose to investigate can therefore have a substantial influence on levels of satisfaction observed. Hall and Dornan (1988) found that average levels of patient satisfaction across studies were much higher where measures focused upon health professionals' humaneness compared to other dimensions such as costs, bureaucracy and attention to psychosocial problems.

Relationships with processes of care

One important test of the validity and, ultimately, the value of measures of patient satisfaction is consideration of the range of aspects of health care that have been shown to influence patients' views. It is important to look for evidence where aspects of health care have been measured independently of patients' views to obtain the most robust evidence ... The following are areas where such robust studies have shown aspects of care to influence patient satisfaction.

Interpersonal skills

How skilled health professionals are in interacting with their patients can substantially influence patient satisfaction. DiMatteo and colleagues (1980) studied 71 doctors working in a New York community hospital. They were asked to perform two experimental tasks. First, they had to judge the emotions portrayed by actors in a film specifically made for the study. Second, they were asked to demonstrate a range of emotions that were then rated by other study participants. Subsequently, patients actually attending the clinics of study doctors were asked to assess independently their doctor's interpersonal skills and technical competence. Doctors' scores for interpreting emotions from, for example, non-verbal cues were found to be significantly related to patients' satisfaction with interpersonal skills but not with technical competence.

Other studies have tried to specify more directly what the interpersonal skills are that are most appreciated by patients. Stiles and colleagues (1979) tape-recorded the consultations of 19 doctors providing general medical care in an American hospital and then subsequently asked their patients to complete a questionnaire about satisfaction with care. Rating scales were used to judge the dialogue between patients and doctors. Patient satisfaction with doctors' interpersonal skills [was] highest when the form of dialogue in consultations was independently assessed from tape-recordings to facilitate the patient in talking about their health problems in their own terms rather than following a rigid closed-ended sequence of medical questions. This approach to consultations is often referred to as a patient-centred style of communication in which questions are asked by the doctor using open-ended questions and the doctor facilitates the expression of patients' concerns and feelings about their presenting problem ...

Information giving

The ability on the part of health professionals to communicate relevant amounts and quality of information to the patient has received particular attention. A meta-analysis of a series of studies in which consultations were independently assessed and patients' views separately elicited after the consultation found that overall information giving had the biggest single effect of all health professional behaviours in influencing patient satisfaction (Roter 1989). This evidence from observational studies is supported from experimental evidence. Ley and Spelman (1967) report a study in which junior doctors in both medical and surgical firms were randomly assigned to communicate with inpatients in one of three ways. In the experimental arm, they were to make a particular effort to elicit patients' concerns. In an attention placebo arm, they were to spend more time communicating with patients but with no particular focus. The control arm involved routine care. In the medical but not the surgical patients, higher satisfaction was reported by patients receiving experimental compared with other forms of communication.

Technical competence

It is often argued from survey evidence that patients may be able competently to judge the interpersonal skills of health professionals but not aspects of technical competence (Sira 1980). To some extent this must be the case since many very technical procedures are performed by health professionals that few patients are sufficiently knowledgeable to evaluate. Nevertheless, there is evidence that patients' views, as expressed in well-designed surveys, may correspond with what health professionals consider appropriate care. Baker (1993) asked 100 patients in each of eight surgeries to complete a satisfaction questionnaire. Their views about the quality and professional standards of the practices were significantly associated with the judgements made by an external professional assessor.

The organization of health care

Patients' views have been shown to correlate with a number of organizational features of their health care. Thus in the Medical Outcomes study, the views of over 17,000 patients were elicited in simple satisfaction questionnaires (Rubin et al. 1996). Patients attending more traditional solo-practitioners rated all aspects of the quality of their care higher than patients attending health maintenance organizations (HMOs). These differences remained after adjustment for patients' demographic and health status characteristics. One immediate consequence of these reactions noted by the investigators was the significantly greater readiness of dissatisfied patients to change their source of health care. Although a number of other studies have suggested that patients are less satisfied in the United States with the newer and somewhat more bureaucratic forms of health care such as HMOs compared to traditional practices, there is also interesting evidence that the longer they stay with new services such as HMOs the more likely it is that levels of satisfaction reach those achieved in more traditional settings (Ross et al. 1981).

Over 7000 patients attending the practices of 126 different GPs were asked to complete a patient satisfaction questionnaire (Baker 1996). The larger the list size, the absence of a personal list system (in which patients register with a named GP) and its being a training practice were all characteristics that decreased patients' expressed satisfaction independently of patients' own characteristics.

Time

It might reasonably be argued that a common denominator of many of the aspects of care that have been shown to have an independent effect on patient satisfaction is the simple parameter of time. It is not surprising that several studies have assessed the effect of this variable. Two studies of British primary care adopted the same basic research design of non-systematic allocation of patients to appointments of varying lengths and used the same patient satisfaction questionnaire as [the] outcome measure (Morrell *et al.* 1986; Ridsdale *et al.* 1989). There was a trend in the direction of longer consultations producing higher levels of patient satisfaction but differences by appointment length were not great and few differences in dimensions of satisfaction were significant. However, in a third study (Howie *et al.* 1991), GPs had some flexibility as to whether patients received a longer consultation compared to the earlier studies in which time was rigidly maintained. In this study, length of consultation was significantly correlated with patient satisfaction, suggesting that when appropriate longer consultations are appreciated.

In this section it has not been the intention to identify the determinants of patient satisfaction, since in almost every field reviewed evidence is still incomplete. Rather it has been shown how wide ranging is the evidence of factors that have been shown by independent measurement to influence patient satisfaction. From this evidence it is clear that accurate assessment of views is essential better to identify aspects of health care appreciated by patients.

Feedback

1 Interpersonal skills affect how well health professionals can interact with their patients and enable them to take an active role in the consultation process. A commitment to good interpersonal skills shows a commitment to respecting patients' dignity. Communication skills are particularly important in showing empathy, assessing the whole range of patients' concerns and in breaking bad news.

2 Information giving allows patients to be intelligently involved in deciding what treatment they will receive. This shows a commitment to respect for their autonomy.

3 Technical competence refers to patients' satisfaction with the professional's ability to deliver appropriate care. This relates to the balance between beneficence and non-maleficence.

4 The organization of health care affects all dimensions of humanity. If patients feel that the process is overly bureaucratic, they may perceive a lack of respect for both dignity and autonomy. For example, they may complain that they feel 'more like a number than a person'. If they cannot see the professional of their choice, they may feel less confident that their treatment is beneficial.

5 Time mainly affects autonomy and dignity. It is difficult to feel valued as an individual (dignity) and as part of the decision-making process (autonomy) during a brief consultation, where there may be pressure on the professional to hurry in order to see the next patient.

Measuring humanity

When evaluating health care, it is essential to decide which aspects of humanity are relevant to the interventions being compared. These will affect your choice of methods for measuring humanity. Activity 13.4 will give you a chance to practise deciding which aspects are the most important for evaluating particular types of intervention.

Activity 13.4

For each of the following health care interventions, write down which aspects of humanity should be evaluated:

1 Introducing immunization against a childhood disease.
2 Inpatient or day case for routine surgery to repair a hernia.
3 Emergency surgery following a road traffic accident.
4 Chemotherapy to treat a life-threatening malignant disease.
5 Long-term rehabilitation of a patient following amputation of a leg.
6 Community care of a patient with long-standing mental illness.
7 Public campaign to encourage smokers to stop smoking.

Feedback

Your answers may be quite different from the following, but you should have considered similar principles:

1 Introducing immunization against a childhood disease:

- autonomy – allowing parents to make an informed choice
- dignity – not undressing the child more than absolutely necessary
- beneficence/non-maleficence – considering the likelihood of children suffering an adverse reaction

2 Inpatient or day case for routine surgery to repair a hernia:

- autonomy – respecting the patient's preference for type of surgery
- dignity would be relevant if you were planning to bring a group of medical students to watch

3 Emergency surgery following a road traffic accident:

- beneficence/non-maleficence – commitment to provide the best treatment without unnecessary tests or procedures; it is possible that dignity and autonomy would be irrelevant for a severely injured patient, however, they should be considered for the family and friends

4 Chemotherapy to treat life-threatening malignant disease:

- autonomy – empowering the patient to be part of the management decision process and respecting their decisions
- dignity – trying to minimize the loss of dignity that often occurs with intensive chemotherapy as patients become nauseated, weak and lose their hair
- beneficence – not pursuing intensive treatment when it is no longer likely to do more good than harm

5 Long-term rehabilitation of a patient following amputation of a leg:

- autonomy – ensuring patient's involvement in planning treatment regimen
- dignity – encouraging patient to maintain appearance and social contacts

6 Community care of a patient with long-standing mental illness:

- dignity – remembering that these are people not just diagnoses, creating a personal environment in facilities
- autonomy – respecting patient's views and decisions; this may be threatened by the illness and aided by appropriate treatment; however, there may be legitimate circumstances where it is appropriate to restrict a patient's autonomy
- non-maleficence – freedom from coercion

7 Public campaign to encourage smokers to stop smoking:

- autonomy – you cannot force this change in behaviour

As you can see, both dignity and autonomy feature in almost every intervention.

Summary

Humanity involves treating people as individuals and respecting their rights of expression and self-determination. It also involves caring for them in a compassionate way and avoiding unnecessary suffering. Four dimensions can be identified. *Autonomy* means respecting (and encouraging) individuals' rights to make choices about their care. *Dignity* means that all individuals are worthy of respect and have the right to be treated with courtesy and with consideration for their feelings. *Beneficence* means striving to provide the intervention which is likely to provide the largest benefit. *Non-maleficence* means avoiding harm, whether caused accidentally or intentionally.

Almost every health care intervention can affect patient autonomy and dignity. When planning an evaluation, you need to consider which dimensions of humanity are most likely to be affected by the interventions that you are evaluating. You should also think about the different areas of the care processes that have been shown to influence patient satisfaction – interpersonal skills, information giving, technical competence, organization of health care and time.

References

Baker R (1993) Use of psychometrics to develop a measure of patient satisfaction for general practice, in Fitzpatrick R and Hopkins A (eds) *Measurement of patients' satisfaction with their care.* London: Royal College of Physicians of London.

Baker R (1996) Characteristics of practices, general practitioners and patients related to levels of patients' satisfaction with consultations. *British Journal of Medical Practice* 46: 601–5.

DiMatteo M, Taranta A, Friedman H and Prince L (1980) Predicting patient satisfaction from physicians' non-verbal communication skills. *Medical Care* 18: 376–87.

Fitzpatrick R (1997) The assessment of patient satisfaction, in Jenkinson C (ed.) *Assessment and evaluation of health and medical care.* Buckingham: Open University Press.

Hall J and Dornan M (1988) Meta-analysis of satisfaction with medical care: description of satisfaction with medical care: a meta-analysis. *Social Science and Medicine* 30: 811–18.

Howie J, Porter M, Heaney D and Hopton J (1991) Long to short consultation ratio: a proxy measure of quality of care for general practice. *British Journal of General Practice* 41: 48–54.

Kmietowicz (2005) Plan aims to end discrimination in mental health services. *British Medical Journal* 330: 113.

Ley P and Spelman M (1967) *Communicating with the patient*. London: Staples Press.

Morrell D, Evans M, Morris R and Roland M (1986) The 'five minute' consultation: effect of time constraint on clinical content and patient satisfaction. *British Medical Journal* 292: 870–2.

Ridsdale L, Carruthers L, Morris R and Ridsdale R (1989) Study of the effect of time availability on the consultation. *Journal of the Royal College of General Practitioners* 39: 488–91.

Ross C, Wheaton B and Duff R (1981) Client satisfaction and the organization of medical practice: why time counts. *Journal of Health and Social Behavior* 22: 243–55.

Roter D (1989) Which facets of communication have strong effects on outcome: a meta analysis, in Stewart M and Roter D (eds) *Communicating with medical patients*. London: Sage.

Rubin H, Gandek B, Rogers W, Kosinski M, McHorney C and Ware J (1996) Patients' ratings of outpatient visits in different practice settings. *Journal of the American Medical Association* 270: 835–40.

Sira ZB (1980) Affective and instrumental components in the physician-patient relationship: an additional component of interaction theory. *Journal of Health and Social Behavior* 21: 170–80.

Stiles W, Putnam S, Wolf M and James S (1979) Interaction exchange structure and patient satisfaction with medical interviews. *Medical Care* 17: 667–79.

Measuring patient satisfaction using quantitative methods

Overview

In the last chapter, you considered what is meant by humanity and how that may be measured in terms of patient satisfaction with the processes of health care. It is possible to use both quantitative methods, such as surveys, and qualitative methods to measure patient satisfaction. In this chapter you will explore the uses of quantitative survey methods in relation to humanity. You will also reconsider the principles of reliability and validity that you learned in Chapter 3.

Learning objectives

By the end of this chapter you should be better able to:

- **explain how a quantitative survey could be used to evaluate patient satisfaction**
- **outline the principal stages of designing a survey**

Key terms

Random sample A group of subjects selected from a population in a random manner (ie each member of the population has an equal chance of being selected).

Sampling frame A list of the members of the population who would be eligible for inclusion in a study.

Health services research and the assessment of humanity

The role of health services research (HSR) in evaluating humanity will vary according to the intervention or service that is being evaluated. HSR may aim to carry out routine monitoring of the general standards of care provided in a specific setting, to evaluate the impact of changes in the method or style of health care provision on the humanity of care, investigate claims of inhumanity/poor standards of care or to understand the reasons for inhumanity and identify ways to improve provision of health care. People's perception of the humanity of care will be shaped by factors such as their sociodemographic characteristics, previous experiences of health care, and also factors such as lifestyle and personality. As the evaluation of humanity is complex it is essential to be clear about which aspects are most relevant, to state precisely the aims of your study and to select appropriate methods to meet these aims. Both quantitative and qualitative methods can be used to evaluate humanity.

When would you use quantitative methods for assessing humanity?

Quantitative methods are most appropriate when you know precisely which aspects of humanity you wish to evaluate. For example, you may wish to assess patient satisfaction with the way that information was provided, or with the hotel services (food, bedding, ward environment) in a hospital. Questionnaires (both psychometric and surveys) are one of the main ways of using quantitative methods for measuring patient satisfaction. Questions are carefully standardized so that they will provide data that can be quantitatively assessed. The participants should be a representative sample of a selected population (such as recipients of a specific form of health care, or sufferers from a particular health condition), and information about them is gathered and analysed systematically.

Before planning your study, it will help to consider the following:

1 *Specificity* – are you investigating a particular intervention (a specific surgical procedure), or making a more general assessment of health care (access to all services in a particular hospital)? This will determine whether you need a narrowly-focused definition of patient satisfaction or to use a broader definition.
2 *Location* – are you examining outpatient, inpatient or health centre care? There will be problems specific to each location.
3 *Timing* – satisfaction changes over time. Patients may forget some of their dissatisfaction after discharge. However, inpatients may feel unable to admit to dissatisfaction. Satisfaction may also change with state of health.
4 *Content* – what aspects of satisfaction are you investigating? The availability of information, the environment or the relationships between people, such as patients and professionals?

The following extract will introduce the principles of surveys. They may be used as investigative tools for a variety of different purposes. In this chapter, you will consider their usefulness for assessing patient satisfaction.

 Activity 14.1

Read the following extract by Layte and Jenkinson (1997) about planning a survey. Consider the following questions:

1 How is a social survey defined?
2 How is a social survey different from an experimental study?

 Social surveys

Social surveys are a method of social research in which investigators attempt to gain a representative sample of a given population, or indeed may sample the entire population, and gain data from self-report. A survey is an investigation in which information is systematically collected, but in which the experimental method is not used (Abramson 1990).

Such a definition, however, tends to refer to a wide number of research methods other than just social surveys such as 'cohort studies' and 'case-control studies'. All of these methods might usefully be grouped under the heading 'observational' studies, as opposed to 'experimental studies' such as the randomized controlled trial . . . More narrowly, the term 'social survey' might be taken to imply surveys of the population, or sub-groups of the population (e.g. people with a particular disease; ethnic minorities; people living in a certain area, etc.), undertaken to gain information on, for example, specific aspects of health, household management, education, employment, etc. It is in this latter sense that 'social survey' is used [here] . . . Data from social surveys tends to be collected in a standardized form that can be coded and analysed statistically. Such data may be gained for the purposes of description and the generation and testing of hypotheses. Consequently, social surveys can be descriptive, or analytic in that they attempt to find the relationship between variables. However, while analytic surveys may attempt to determine the association of variables, or may, in longitudinal designs, attempt to determine the effect of a certain event, individuals are not randomly assigned to groups and consequently the study is observational rather than truly experimental. Some established texts in the field assume that analytic surveys are experimental by nature (see, for example, Oppenheim 1966, 1992) but given there is no assignment of cases to groups this is unlikely to ever be the case . . .

Planning a survey

Carrying out a survey can seem a relatively straightforward undertaking, requiring good organizational skills and some common sense. However, while it is probably fair to assume that most people could, given the appropriate level of funding, send out any number of questionnaires, the development of a properly conducted survey requires more than simply an ability to seal envelopes, or ask people questions! Appropriate questions have to be developed and piloted, or standardized questionnaires chosen; sampling techniques need to be considered in order to gain as representative a sample as possible and the issue of the mode of administration and its possible effect needs to be carefully considered.

 Feedback

1 The authors of this passage define surveys as studies which obtain self-report data from a population (or a representative sample) for the purpose of gaining information on specific aspects of health.

2 A survey is unlikely to be able to achieve random allocation of cases whereas an experimental study should always randomly allocate cases.

Layte and Jenkinson (1997) identify a number of steps that should be followed in a quantitative study that uses a survey or questionnaire. An adapted version of these stages is considered in more detail in the next section.

Stages in survey design

In this section we will use the example of a survey study to investigate patient satisfaction to consider the stages in turn. It is not always necessary, however, to perform all the stages cited.

Stage 1: select a topic and review the relevant literature

This is an essential step in performing any research.

Stage 2: develop a set of issues to be addressed by the survey

The issues to be addressed are those aspects of humanity that you wish to assess, such as how well patients are empowered to play an active role in making decisions about their treatment. The reading by Fitzpatrick (1997) in Chapter 13 suggested 11 domains that might contribute to patient satisfaction (Table 13.1). Each of these could be assessed by items in a questionnaire. If you are developing a psychometric instrument, the conceptual domains that the questionnaire is intended to address are sometimes described as a conceptual framework (see Stage 4 below).

Stage 3: identify the population to be surveyed

The population is defined in terms of its experience of the health care intervention that you are evaluating. However, unless you can survey all members of this population, you will need to *select* an appropriate sample (see Stage 9).

Stage 4: develop a conceptual framework

This is particularly important if you are developing a psychometric questionnaire (where you will add up all the questions to form a single score), but it may also be useful for survey-type questionnaires. A conceptual framework describes all the relevant aspects of the construct that you want to measure. The development of the conceptual framework should be based on relevant literature, consultation with experts, review of other existing questionnaires and possibly qualitative interviews with patients. Identifying a conceptual framework of patient satisfaction is complex and as yet there is no universal consensus about the contributing domains (Crow *et al.* 2002). There is also some debate as to whether the domains of patient satisfaction can be combined into a single overall score representing a unitary concept (Carr-Hill 1992). Sitzia and Wood (1997) provide a useful review of a number of conceptual models that have been proposed.

Stage 5: draft a questionnaire (or identify an existing questionnaire)

If there is already an instrument that addresses all of the aspects that you want to measure, then use this instead. There is no point in reinventing the wheel. Drafting a new questionnaire can be difficult. Assuming that a new questionnaire is necessary you need to develop questions that measure each of the relevant aspects of patient satisfaction that you have identified in your conceptual framework. You also need to decide how these questions are to be administered – for example, by self-completion questionnaire (which could be sent in the post) or interviewer administered questionnaire.

Activity 14.2 will briefly mention the principles behind choosing questions and administering them.

 Activity 14.2

Read the extract by Stone (1993) below about designing questionnaires. Consider the following:

1   What are the features of a 'good' question?
2   What factors would you need to take into account when deciding the format of the questionnaire?

 A good questionnaire is one that works

When a questionnaire is administered to a potential respondent an elaborate and subtle process is started which is intended to end in the transmission of useful and accurate information from the respondent to the inquirer. Consider what this process involves. A question or series of questions have to be posed in a clear, comprehensible, and appropriate manner so that the respondent can formulate, articulate, and transmit the answers effectively. These answers must be recorded, coded, and analysed without bias, errors, or misrepresentation of the respondent's views. A well designed questionnaire ensures the smooth unfolding of this chain of events from start to finish.

What are the characteristics of a well designed questionnaire? There is no hard and fast answer. A good questionnaire is one that works. In other words, it is self validating. Nevertheless, there are several criteria which should be met in advance of unleashing a questionnaire on an unsuspecting public. Some of these may seem blindingly obvious, but it is surprising how often they appear to have been overlooked in practice . . .

An *appropriate* questionnaire is one which is capable of providing answers to the questions being asked. There is no point, for example, in asking a pathologist how he establishes a rapport with his patients, or a general practitioner what time he starts his ward round.

An *intelligible* question is one which the respondent can understand. This means using language that the respondent uses. I recently encountered a survey on the sequelae of circumcision which required mothers to choose one of a series of carefully worded statements. The statements were in English and the respondents were mostly first generation Urdu speaking immigrants.

An *unambiguous* question is one which means the same to both the respondent and the inquirer. If you ask a mixed group of psychoanalysts and statisticians to define what they understand by the term 'regression analysis' you will receive dramatically divergent answers.

A question may appear *unbiased* until you try to interpret the answers. The objective is to ensure that you are no more likely to trigger one kind of response than another. I used to marvel at the naivety of a certain country's immigration department, who insisted on asking that old music hall joke of a question 'Are you or have you ever been a member of the Communist party?' A less obvious source of bias is the dependence on the memory of the respondent who may remember certain events in a highly selective fashion. This is called recall bias. An example of this is the attempt to establish the cause of a birth defect by asking mothers whether anything untoward occurred during the pregnancy.

A question should be *omnicompetent* – capable of coping with all possible responses. In reality that is an impossible expectation of any question since the range of potential answers is limited only by the number of people who might answer the questionnaire. We should try, however, to anticipate most of them including a category 'Other' or leaving space for comments. The response most frequently overlooked in designing a multioption question is 'don't know' particularly when a 'yes/no' answer is being sought. Human uncertainty and indecisiveness may be an irritating inconvenience but it cannot be ignored.

The *coding* system must be carefully checked for ambiguity and overlap. The rule here is that the categories should be exhaustive but mutually exclusive. Thus if ages are being split into 10 year bands it must be clear which bands the ages on the boundaries – 20, 30, 40, etc. – lie in. Ideally, the answers should be self-coding, both to save time and resources when the data have to be computerised and to eliminate a source of errors.

A questionnaire should always be *piloted* before use. This has two purposes: to iron out any design faults which have been missed (and there are always a surprising number) and to enable a formal evaluation to be performed . . .

Finally, a questionnaire should be *ethical*. Until recently, ethics committees took no real interest in surveys which did not use invasive or hazardous procedures. Nowadays they regard research as potentially harmful even if it consists of a single question. They will need reassurance about the necessity for the investigation, its scientific rigour, the sensitivity with which it is conducted, and obtaining of informed consent from the subjects.

So much for theory. Now for the practical task of sitting down and creating your questionnaire. If you have never done it (and even if you have) the prospect can be intimidating. Here is a list of steps you can take to try to achieve your goal quickly and easily. It is not a recipe for success but it may help you avoid disaster . . .

Designing a questionnaire

(1) Decide what data you need
(2) Select items for inclusion
(3) Design individual questions
(4) Compose wording
(5) Design layout
(6) Think about coding
(7) Prepare first draft and pretest
(8) Pilot and evaluate

(9) Perform survey
(10) Start again!

The format of the questions depends largely on how the survey will be performed – by post, direct interview, or telephone and whether the data are quantitative or qualitative. For qualitative research, open rather than closed questions may be more appropriate. Open questions are also useful for the predesign stage of a project, when you are trying to decide what data you need (step 1 above). Closed questions may prompt dichotomous responses (usually yes/no) or take the form of alternative statements, a checklist, or a rating scale. The choice of a question or scale will also depend on whether the variable being measured can be expressed categorically (for example, religion) or continuously (for example, blood pressure). Avoid the temptation to force responses into a categorical mould since many health variables, including those relating to non-biological factors such as emotions, can be adequately described only along a continuum. A popular means of recording an opinion is the Likert scale, in which the respondent is given a statement and is asked to tick one of the categories: strongly agree, agree, no opinion, disagree, strongly disagree.

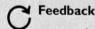

Feedback

1 Think about Stone's five criteria for survey questions:

- Appropriate = asking the right thing.
- Intelligible = easy to understand.
- Unambiguous = meaning what you want the question to mean and nothing else.
- Unbiased = covering the issues consistently for all health care interventions.
- Omnicompetent = able to record any response that the subject could make.

2 In a survey, questions may be open – 'What did you like about the food?' – or closed – 'Did you like the food?'. Open questions require the respondent to write a text answer and may elicit more varied responses, but can be difficult to analyse. For closed questions, respondents are often asked to indicate their answers using a rating scale (e.g. always/often/sometimes/never). It may be necessary to develop a response scale that is appropriate to the population being investigated. For example, when asking children how they feel, you might show a picture of a series of faces ranging from sad to happy and ask which one represents their feelings best. Patients who have communication difficulties may need a questionnaire that is phrased very simply or perhaps that can be read out loud by an interviewer. In some situations – for example, people with dementia – it may not be possible to ask the patient themselves and it may be necessary to ask a proxy on their behalf. The importance of choosing an appropriate proxy was discussed in Chapter 3. There is some evidence to suggest that proxy respondents report greater dissatisfaction than patients themselves would (Walker and Restuccia 1984).

How the items in a questionnaire are phrased and presented can be very important in minimizing response bias. This is discussed in more detail below.

Stage 6: pre-test or pilot the questionnaire

This is an essential step that is often missed out. The draft questionnaire should be administered to a group of people similar to those who will eventually be part of the sample. The questionnaire should be administered in a face-to-face interview. Pre-testing helps to make sure that all the important aspects have been covered (content validity), to identify problem questions that are difficult to answer, to suggest improved wording of questions that are not clear and to estimate completion time. Respondents can also be asked if they have any other comments to make about the questionnaire. Pre-test interviews can be audio-taped to ensure that you have a good record of what is said. The draft questionnaire should then be revised in the light of the data from the pre-test to form a final version.

Stage 7: finalize the questionnaire

Stages 1–6 will enable you to develop a questionnaire. If the questionnaire is a psychometric one, you will then need to ensure that it is reliable and valid. This might be done using two stages of field testing. In the preliminary field test you might conduct item analyses to identify the questions with the best psychometric properties. This is known as *item reduction*. Having eliminated the poorest questions, you would then develop a shorter version of the questionnaire which you would test in a second field test. This final field test will evaluate the extent to which the questionnaire is reliable, valid and responsive. You might like to look back at this chapter to remind yourself of these concepts.

Stage 8: select an appropriate sample of the population

It is important that the individuals who are included in your sample actually represent the population to which you wish to apply your results. Sampling refers to the process of identifying individuals for inclusion in your survey. Selection of individuals may involve either random or non-random sampling techniques.

Activity 14.3 will consider sampling as it applies to survey studies.

Activity 14.3

Read the following extract by Layte and Jenkinson (1997) that describes random sampling and then answer the following questions:

1 What processes are necessary in order to perform random sampling?
2 What are the advantages of systematic sampling compared with simple random sampling?
3 What are the advantages of cluster sampling?

📖 Random sampling

Sampling is an important aspect of successful survey research. If the sample is not representative of the population from which it is drawn then the results gained from it cannot be generalized to the population level. The most commonly adopted method of sampling is known as 'probability sampling' in which each person in the population has a known probability of being selected. Random sampling is the most familiar form of probability sampling, and is a technique whereby each sampling unit (e.g. an individual person) will have the same probability of being selected. When used without qualification random sampling is often referred to as 'simple random sampling'. Random sampling requires the following process: first, a sampling frame must be selected. This is usually a list containing all the people from which the sample is to be selected. Such a list may be all those people registered to vote in a given area or all those people registered with general practitioners in a given area. However, despite the fact one would hope that everyone in the country was accurately entered on electoral registers and general practice lists, the names that appear on a list rarely reflect the population perfectly accurately. They are often out of date, containing names of people who have moved out of the area or who have died. Furthermore, others will have moved into the area but not yet registered themselves on the electoral register or with doctors, and still others will not appear on such lists because they are homeless, never visit a doctor, have not replied to communications about their name and address, and so on. Ideally, some check should be done on the data in the sampling frame to determine that it is at least representative of the population it is meant to reflect. After the sampling frame has been selected, then the sample size should be determined. This is not an easy task, especially in those instances where power calculations (which indicate the ability of a study to determine relationships between variables being measured) cannot be made as there are no prior hypotheses about, for example, possible differences between certain groups of the population on a given variable or variables (see below). Pragmatically, most social survey research projects try to ascertain the largest sample that can be gained with the resources available. Once the sample size has been determined, subjects are selected at random, usually from tables of random numbers, or using computer programs that generate random numbers.

Another form of probability sampling is 'systematic sampling'. Once the first case has been randomly selected the choice of all others is predetermined. A systematic sample is one gained by taking every '*nth*' subject in a list containing the population to be sampled. Consequently, not all members of the population have the same chance of being selected for inclusion in the sample. Once the sample size as a percentage of the population, or 'sampling fraction', has been decided the random selection of the starting point determines the whole sample. Systematic sampling is likely to produce a more even spread of the sample over the population than does simple random sampling. This can lead to greater precision than does simple random sampling in those instances where the sample is ordered in some systematic way (e.g. by age). One particular problem of this sampling method concerns instances where the sampling interval coincides with some periodic interval in the list, but such periodicals are rare and generally easy to detect (Moser and Kalton 1972).

In instances where simple random or systematic sampling would create a sample too geographically spread then a method known as cluster sampling can be adopted. Cluster sampling is a method for gaining a sample from a population in two stages. This method takes advantage of the fact that most populations are structured in some way. For example, all people registered to vote constitute the national electorate. If this group is to act as the primary sampling frame it is possible to select a random group of local constituencies. Random sampling is used to select out groups to be included at the second stage and, technically, all subjects included in the selected samples are then surveyed. The advantage of this method is that it produces, as the name suggests, 'clusters' of respondents, thereby reducing interviewing and travelling costs. Cluster sampling is effectively a special case of 'multi-stage' sampling in which successive samples are taken. Thus, the national electorate may constitute the sampling frame, from which a random selection of local constituencies are selected, from which a random selection of local wards are drawn and, potentially, from which a random selection of respondents are chosen. Both cluster and multi-stage sampling increase the chance of sampling error with each stage in the process. Sampling error refers to inaccuracies in inferences about a population that have been derived from a sample survey. Thus, if a multi-stage sample selects more constituencies in the North of England than the South then the results are likely to reflect the views *of* people in the North rather than the South. The chance *of* such sampling error occurring increases substantially when samples are small.

It is possible that where a researcher wishes to compare sub-groups of the population, one or other of the groups is under-represented. To avoid this problem researchers can select samples of equal size within each of the groups. For example, one may wish to compare the attitudes to treatment of male and female heart attack survivors. However, a random sample would produce more men than women, given that heart attack is more common in males. Consequently, one may decide not to sample from the group as a whole, but to select random samples of equal size from the two sub-groups.

 Feedback

1 Random sampling requires the definition of a sampling frame (a list of all those eligible to be included); analysis of the data in the sampling frame to determine whether it really represents the population to be studied (e.g. analysing the age or social class structure of the sample to see whether it represents the population); and estimation of the sample size required.

2 Systematic sampling produces a more even spread across the population compared with simple random sampling. However, this can be a problem if there is a periodic relationship between individuals.

3 Cluster sampling can reduce travelling and interviewing time as it can produce a sample that is geographically clustered. However, cluster sampling is likely to increase sampling error.

Non-random sampling

It is not always possible to perform random sampling. The text below describes two alternatives.

Opportunistic sampling describes the process of including those individuals who are conveniently accessible. It may be the only practical technique if time and resources are limited. However, there is no reason to believe that the subjects represent the wider population. It may be necessary to compare a number of key attributes in the sample with those in the reference population to determine how representative the sample is.

Snowball sampling refers to the practice of identifying some individuals (by any technique) and asking them to nominate more individuals who might also be willing to take part in the study. This is a useful technique where the subject is particularly sensitive, because the nominated individuals are more likely to agree to take part than other members of the public. However, those who respond may not be representative of the wider population. As they have been nominated (often by their friends), they may have many characteristics in common with those who nominated them and their replies may tend to be similar. This can be a source of bias.

An important feature of sampling is estimation of sample size. Although you may be able to estimate sample size statistically, it is often necessary to simply survey as many as possible.

Stage 9: train interviewers (if necessary)

If your survey requires interviewers, it is important to train them to ask questions in a consistent fashion. If at all possible, they should be kept unaware of which intervention their interviewees have experienced. As was discussed in Chapter 5, this is described as blinding. It is essential that the interviewers treat those who have received different interventions in the same way to avoid bias.

Stage 10: collect data

The timing of data collection may be very important. Remember that bias may be a problem if you survey patients a long time after they have experienced the intervention (see Chapter 5). Responses will need to be coded in a way that facilitates analysis.

Stage 11: perform analyses and write reports

It is important to decide how you will treat non-response and missing data. These are covered briefly in Activity 14.4.

Bias in questionnaires

There are several sources of bias that can affect questionnaire responses when measuring patient satisfaction. 'Framing effects' refer to how responses are affected by how the question is phrased and information in preceding questions (Kahneman and Tversky 1984). Ensuring that questions are easy to understand, unambiguous and appropriate can help to reduce framing effects as can separating questions that may influence each other. 'Acquiescence bias' or 'yea-saying' (Couch and Keniston 1960) describes the tendency of patients to agree regardless of the question intent. This can be a particular problem with respect to patient satisfaction as patients may be unwilling to admit to dissatisfaction with the care they have received. In patient satisfaction studies, acquiescent response is most likely to occur in respondents who are older, more ill, less educated and have lower income. Acquiescence can be minimized by including a balance of both positively and negatively phrased questions.

The timing and mode of administration of questionnaires can also affect the results of patient satisfaction results. Crow *et al.* (2002) report that in general questionnaires administered in person result in more satisfaction being reported. This tends to be attributed to patients wanting to give an answer that is socially acceptable. The same review indicates that questionnaires that are administered face to face or by telephone have higher response rates than those administered by post. If non-response is high then there is a danger that the group who do not respond is systematically different from the group who do respond and this introduces bias into the results of the study. Incentives such as reminders and pre-paid reply envelopes can help to reduce the rate of non-response. However, even in studies with a very good response rate there will inevitably be some missing data as respondents will sometimes miss out a question. There are some well-established methods for dealing with missing data. For example, the developers of the SF-36 (Ware *et al.* 1993) have a specific algorithm which they recommend for imputing missing data with this questionnaire, provided a minimum amount has been completed. In general, imputation methods should be used with caution (Layte and Jenkinson 1997).

 Activity 14.4

Now that you have considered sources of bias in patient satisfaction questionnaires, consider the following questions:

1 What might be the effects of acquiescence bias in a patient satisfaction survey?
2 Why is non-response potentially a problem in surveys?
3 How might you reduce the extent of non-response?
4 How can missing data be addressed at the analysis stage?

 Feedback

1 Acquiescence bias would result in respondents tending to agree with the question. If the questions were phrased positively, then this form of bias would result in a higher degree of satisfaction being reported than was actually experienced. If the questions were phrased both positively and negatively, acquiescent respondents would still tend to agree with the question, but they would agree equally with positive and negative questions and the effects should balance out. However, this form of bias would still be a problem if survey questions were analysed individually.

2 Non-respondents may be systematically different to respondents (e.g. they may have a different level of education or social class). This may influence the results of the study.

3 Non-response can be reduced by providing pre-paid envelopes, appropriate covering letters and small inducements to complete the questionnaire.

4 It is sometimes possible to impute missing data. However, this should be performed with caution and using an existing well-tested algorithm.

Summary

Quantitative methods of assessing patient satisfaction are appropriate when you know precisely which aspects of humanity you wish to evaluate. When planning a survey, you should consider the following points:

1 *Specificity of the survey* – are you investigating a particular intervention (e.g. a specific surgical procedure), or making a more general assessment of health care (such as access to all services in a particular hospital)? This will determine whether you need a narrowly-focused definition of patient satisfaction, or whether you should include satisfaction with several different issues.
2 *Location of survey* – are you examining outpatient, inpatient or health centre care? There will be problems specific to each location.
3 *Timing of survey* – satisfaction changes over time. Patients may forget some of their dissatisfaction after discharge. However, inpatients may feel unable to admit to lack of satisfaction. Satisfaction may also change with state of health.
4 *Content* – which aspects of satisfaction are you investigating? Are you investigating the availability of information, or the environment or the relationships between people such as patients and professionals?

The chapter has also guided you through the various stages in conducting a survey. There is the same need to avoid bias and confounding in surveys as in other study designs.

References

Abramson JH (1990) *Survey methods in community medicine*. Edinburgh: Churchill Livingstone.

Carr-Hill RA (1992) The measurement of patient satisfaction. *Journal of Public Health Medicine* 14: 236–49.

Couch A and Keniston K (1960) Yeasayers and naysayers: agreeing response set as a personality variable. *Journal of Abnormal and Social Psychology* 60: 151–74.

Crow R, Gage H, Hampson S, Hart J, Kimber A, Storey L *et al.* (2002) The measurement of satisfaction with healthcare: implications for practice from a systematic review of the literature. *Health Technology Assessment* 6: 32.

Fitzpatrick R (1997) The assessment of patient satisfaction, in Jenkinson C (ed.) *Assessment and evaluation of health and medical care*. Buckingham: Open University Press.

Kahneman D and Tversky A (1984) Choices, values and frames. *American Psychologist* 39: 341–50.

Layte R and Jenkinson C (1997) Social surveys, in Jenkinson C (ed.) *Assessment and evaluation of health and medical care*. Buckingham: Open University Press.

Moser CA and Kalton G (1972) *Survey methods in social investigation*. London: Heinemann Educational.

Oppenheim B (1966) *Questionnaire design and attitude measurement*. New York: Basic Books.

Oppenheim B (1992) *Questionnaire design, interviewing and attitude measurement*. London: Pinter.

Sitzia J and Wood N (1997) Patient satisfaction: a review of issues and concepts. *Social Science and Medicine* 45: 1829–43.

Stone DH (1993) Design and questionnaire. *British Medical Journal* 307: 1264–6.

Walker A and Restuccia J (1984) Obtaining information on patient satisfaction with hospital care: mail versus telephone. *Health Services Research* 19: 291–306.

Ware JE, Snow KK, Kosinski M and Gandek B (1993) *The SF36 health survey manual and interpretation guide*. Boston, MA: The Health Institute, New England Medical Center.

15 Measuring patient satisfaction using qualitative methods

Overview

In the last chapter, you considered how quantitative survey methods could be used to evaluate humanity. In this chapter you will consider the use of qualitative methods to do the same.

Learning objectives

By the end of this chapter you should be better able to:

- **describe a variety of qualitative methods that could be used to evaluate humanity**
- **describe the advantages and disadvantages of various qualitative methods**
- **make an informed choice about methods to evaluate humanity**

Key terms

Ethnography A research method used in sociology and anthropology that systematically describes the culture of a group of people.

Focus group A group interview including between 6 and 12 participants and a facilitator who guides the discussion to cover the research topics.

Hawthorne effect The tendency for the act of observing behaviour to change the behaviour that is being observed.

Nominal group technique A method of developing group consensus recorded in which participants first record their individual views on the topic, views are then discussed and then recorded privately again by each participant.

Participant observation Method of data collection in which the researcher participates in the process that is being studied, as well as acting as observer.

When would you use qualitative methods for assessing humanity?

Qualitative methods are concerned with how people behave and how social systems operate. In other words, they are focused on individuals rather than on diseases or clinical outcomes. They are ideal techniques for evaluating humanity when you are unable to decide in advance which aspects are most important in a particular situation. Qualitative methods enable you to learn what people do, explore the way they interpret their experiences, and also to examine the impact that the research process has on their behaviour. These methods seek to discover why individuals hold particular beliefs and why they perform particular actions.

Sometimes qualitative methods are used to help plan a quantitative study. For example, you may wish to use an RCT to compare two health interventions. You could use qualitative methods to determine which health care outcomes are important to patients, then design your RCT to measure these outcomes. It is also possible to use qualitative methods to explore issues or problems identified in quantitative studies. For example, a quantitative survey may have identified that patients are dissatisfied with the way nurses speak to them. You could then use qualitative methods to investigate the reasons for this behaviour.

Types of qualitative method

There are two main types of qualitative method that may be useful in health care evaluation: observation and in-depth interviews.

Observation

Observation techniques seek to examine what people do as well as what they say. Qualitative observation may be non-participant or participant. It may also be covert or overt. These differing types of qualitative observation are described below.

Non-participant observation

This describes the process of visiting one or more places where health care is occurring and observing what patients (and staff) do and say. For example, if you want to measure patients' satisfaction with their experiences in an outpatient department, you could simply visit the department, sit down, watch how people behave and listen to their conversations.

Participant observation

This is a method of data collection where the researcher participates in the process that is being studied, as well as acting as observer. For example, the researcher might be working as a nurse but also conducting observation of the ward. This dual role is difficult to achieve and there are important ethical considerations as the participants are usually unaware that they are being observed. Patient satisfaction could be observed and examined by watching how patients react to a variety of aspects of the health care process. If patients are reasonably well but do not eat their food, this may indicate that they are not satisfied with its quality (even if they claim that it is satisfactory).

Covert observation

This refers to the situation where the people being observed are unaware of the observer. Covert participant observation involves the researcher becoming part of the group (staff or patient) without allowing those observed to know that they are being studied. Covert non-participant observation refers to a situation where the researcher simply watches without being noticed (through a one-way mirror, perhaps). Covert research may raise some ethical issues, but sometimes this approach may be justifiable.

Overt observation

This occurs when the subjects are aware that they are being observed.

Activity 15.1 considers some of the features of observational research. The related extract refers to 'ethnographic' research. This is a research methodology, associated with sociology and anthropology, that systematically describes the culture of a group of people.

 Activity 15.1

Read the following extract from Ziebland and Wright (1997) about using observational methods. As you read, try to answer the following questions:

1 What are the differences between participant and non-participant observation?
2 What are the principal features of:

    a) covert observation?
    b) overt observation?

3 Can you think of reasons why you might be denied access to patients and to some parts of the health care process?

 Observational methods

While there are questionnaire designs and interviewing techniques which may help to minimize the disparity between what people do and what they say they do, a description of occurrences in a natural setting tells a more convincing story than is possible when relying on questionnaire responses alone. This advantage of observational research methods is all the more applicable if the researcher is conducting their research *in cognito*, as a covert participant observer. If the subjects are aware that they are being observed they may alter their behaviour, perhaps from increased self-consciousness, or to present themselves in a favourable light; or to adhere to official rules of comportment. Some classic research in health settings has been conducted by 'under cover' researchers who gained access by working as staff, e.g. Goffman's (1961) study which was undertaken while he was working in a mental hospital (as an assistant to the athletic director). Having an additional role to perform, especially if the researcher is 'undercover', will inevitably sometimes interfere with the process of data collection, but may be the only way to achieve naturalistic observations in the setting of interest . . .

Posing as a patient in a mental hospital may be an even more extreme covert role than taking a job of work to gain access to a research environment. A controversial use of the pseudo patient in a research study is Rosenhan's work 'On being sane in insane places' (1973), which described the diagnostic and subsequent experiences of eight 'sane' people who gained secret admission to psychiatric hospitals. All presented with the same symptoms, the complaint that they were hearing voices. None was recognized as an impostor and, despite behaving in a 'normal' and cooperative manner and not complaining of symptoms again after admittance, the average length of time to discharge was 19 days, with a range from seven to 52 days. Unsurprisingly, the covert nature of Rosenhan's work did nothing to endear him (or the wider research community) to the profession of psychiatry. Covert participant observation has rather fallen from favour because of the difficult ethical issues involved. There are often ethical problems if researchers pose as health care workers or patients. There may be additional concerns about the misuse of resources if the deception continues long-term. The other end of the observation spectrum is overt and non-participant observation, where the role of the researcher is acknowledged and the aim is to impact as little as possible on the setting. When observations are conducted in an overt and non-participant manner, it may be argued that the longer the observer is present in the setting (or the less informed are the subjects about the true purpose of the research) the more naturalistic will be the observations. Strong, as a non-participant observer, by conducting 'fly on the wall' research on hundreds of paediatric consultations in Britain and the United States, was able to detail the complex rules which make up the institutionalized roles of patients and doctors (Strong 1979) . . .

Lofland observes that many ethnographies have arisen from the researcher's personal biography (Lofland and Lofland 1984). Observations may be overt or covert, participant or non-participant. Some aspects of the research role will be eased through familiarity with the setting, although the dangers of 'going native' may be all the more acute. Barrie Thorne was an antiwar activist when the fieldwork for 'Protest and the problem of credibility' was conducted and Julius Roth was a patient in a tuberculosis hospital when he did the fieldwork for his study 'Timetables: structuring the passage of time in hospital treatment and other careers' (Roth 1963). While the qualitative researcher may see the research possibilities of an extended illness episode, such opportunities are unlikely to be actively sought.

Gaining access

Negotiating access to the naturalistic research setting is a vital part of ethnographic observation. Settings which are likely to be of interest to the health researcher are rarely characterized by entirely open access. A waiting room in an out-patients' department or GPs surgery is certainly an environment with less restricted access arrangements than an operating theatre, but observations which are curtailed on the public side of the clinician's door will have a limited scope. Failed research is rarely reported and many ethnographic research projects may have ground to a halt or veered off on a 'path of least resistance' (Lee 1993) as a result of difficulties which occur when trying to gain access. Dowell comments that it is an area of social dynamics which is worthy of research in itself (Dowell et al. 1996). Access will need to be negotiated at the appropriate levels within the hierarchy and at each gatekeeping encounter it may be necessary to accept the imposition of conditions on the research. These may involve methodological restrictions; the negotiation of a reciprocal arrangement where access is allowed on the condition that the gatekeeper's research agenda is (also) addressed; and an agreement that the gatekeeper has the final say in any resultant publications (Lee 1993). It should be noted that while gatekeepers in relatively powerful positions are able to impose restrictions in an overt manner, those at other levels in the hierarchy may be even more effective in scuppering the process if they have not been appropriately consulted or if the researcher antagonizes staff whose cooperation is essential . . .

Once access has been achieved, the importance of establishing (and deserving) the trust of participants in the research setting cannot be over-emphasized. If rich data is to be gained it is important that investigators act in a manner which will maximize the information which is made available to them. Lofland discusses ways in which the problems of 'getting along' may be minimized with regard to stance and style. The stance which most fieldworkers take is, they suggest, 'trust combined with a healthy dose of scepticism'. In many situations the researcher's style will be successful if it combines a non-threatening demeanour with what the authors describe as a display of 'socially acceptable incompetence' (Lofland and Lofland 1984).

↻ Feedback

1 Participant observation involves the researcher being a part of the process that is being studied. In theory, a researcher who is accepted as a normal part of the care process will be ideally placed to observe all aspects of care and patient behaviour. This depends on the researcher having adequate access to patients, staff and all relevant locations. Non-participant observation involves the researcher in simply being present and alert to what is occurring. In theory, if researchers are present for long enough, patients and staff will start to ignore them and behave in their usual manner.

2 Some advantages and disadvantages of covert versus overt observation are these:

a) Covert observation has the advantage of not influencing the normal behaviour of the subjects. However, it requires that the researcher's status is concealed. This limits the observer's ability to ask questions that could help to understand the observed behaviour. It may be considered unethical to observe subjects as part of a study without asking their permission.

b) Overt observation has the advantage of allowing the researcher to question the subjects. It can also avoid ethical problems because it is easier to obtain informed consent from subjects who know that they are being observed. The main disadvantage of overt observation is the tendency for people to change their behaviour when they know they are being studied. This is described as the Hawthorne effect.

3 Be aware of the importance of gaining access to the appropriate parts of the health care process – that is, to patients, staff and important locations. You may experience restrictions imposed by individuals who feel that your research could threaten patient welfare or their own practice. Members of staff may not have enough time or space to accommodate a researcher. If they are concerned that the quality of their practice is substandard, they may wish to conceal this from you. It may be helpful to make audio or video recordings. However, this requires the consent of those who will be recorded.

Interviews

Interviews differ from observation because they involve specific communication between the researcher and subjects, outside subjects' normal behaviour. Interviews may be described according to their degree of structure. A highly structured interview may involve the researcher asking a predetermined set of questions in a predetermined order, whereas a semi-structured interview may be no more than a conversation about a series of predetermined topics. Interviews may also be described according to the number of people interviewed at any one time. They may be individual interviews or group interviews. Activity 15.2 examines some alternative forms of group interview.

Activity 15.2

Read the following extract from Ziebland and Wright (1997) that describes focus groups and nominal groups. While you are reading, think about how a nominal group is different from a focus group and when each might be used.

Focus groups

'A focus group is a carefully planned discussion designed to obtain perceptions on a defined area of interest in a permissive, non-threatening environment' (Krueger 1994: 6). Typically, this involves six to 12 participants in each group in at least three groups the members of which come together in a 'focused' discussion of the topic.

Although focus groups originated in social science (Merton and Kendall 1946) until recently their use has been largely limited to market research (Morgan 1988; Fontana and Frey 1994). More recently still, focus groups have found favour among health and health services researchers to examine people's experiences of disease and of health services and to explore attitudes and needs of staff (Kitzinger 1995) . . .

Nominal groups

Nominal Group Technique (NGT) is a method for structuring small group meetings that allows individual judgements about a topic or issue to be pooled effectively and used in situations in which uncertainty or disagreement exists about the nature of a problem and possible solutions (Moore 1994).

The technique is useful in identifying problems, exploring solutions and establishing priorities (Moore 1994). In health related research it has been used as a way of dealing with conflicting scientific evidence . . . Typically, the nominal group meeting is structured in seven stages. First, participants write down their views on the topic. Second, each then gives one of these views to the facilitator who records it on a flip chart. Third, the written suggestions are grouped where similar and discussed by the group. Next, each member of the group ranks each idea. The rankings are then presented to the group, after which the overall ranking is discussed and reranked. Lastly, the final rankings are tabulated and fed back to the group. This voting procedure can give the impression that the final result indicates group consensus, but usually the main outcome is the generation of ideas (Moore 1994).

Feedback

A focus group comprises between 6 and 12 participants and a facilitator. The participants often share similar characteristics, such as clinical diagnosis or ethnic type. The facilitator guides the discussion to cover the research topics. Because the process is a group discussion, participants may feel able to express feelings and ideas that they would not mention in an individual interview. Once one participant has expressed dissatisfaction with a health service, others may feel more able to do so. The group interaction may help the researcher understand how knowledge and opinions are formed through social interaction.

A nominal group is similar to a focus group, but concentrates on one topic. It is therefore more useful for situations when it is the topic rather than the group process that is of interest (Jones and Hunter 1995). There is a more rigid structure, with participants expressing their individual views on the topic. These views are grouped and discussed by the whole group. Each participant then privately ranks each idea and a group view of the ideas, in order of importance, is produced.

Interviews can be used for a variety of purposes in relation to health care evaluation. Ziebland and Wright (1997) provide a useful overview. They suggest that qualitative interviews could be used to form preliminary studies, to explore sensitive topics, to further investigate the meaning and understanding of particular concepts, and to further explore ideas that arise from other quantitative work. All of these might be relevant to aspects of humanity.

Validity of qualitative methods

In Chapter 3 you examined reliability and validity as they apply to quantitative methods. It is just as important that qualitative methods are reliable and valid. The reliability and validity of the method used depends on the following factors being appropriate for the question that is being studied:

- study design;
- sampling method;
- method of collecting data;
- method of analysing data.

Study design, sampling and data collection will be examined in the following activity (analysis of qualitative data is considered in the next section).

 Activity 15.3

Read the following extract from Ziebland and Wright (1997) and consider how study design, sampling and data collection can help to maximize reliability and validity.

Maximising reliability and validity design

The methods which are used should be appropriate to the research question. Very broadly, if the question is of the 'how often' variety, a quantitative method will be needed, while 'why' and 'what' and 'how', exploring process and subjective meanings, is the main purpose of qualitative methods (Pope and Mays 1995). However, too blunt a distinction can be misleading since counting is sometimes an entirely appropriate feature of an ethnographic study and surveys can certainly be designed to address complex causal relationships.

Sampling

Sample selection is important in qualitative research, even though the object of the study is not to generate statistically significant findings. While it is not relevant to use power calculations to determine the size of the sample, there are requirements appropriate to the aims of the research. Sampling will sometimes be conducted to provide as broad a range as possible, according to the researchers' understanding of factors which might affect the observations or the perspective of individual or group interviewees. These may include the type of institution; whether a rural or urban location; the sex, age and ethnic group of respondents and so on.

Where interviews are conducted in a group, particular attention should be paid to the composition of the sample for each group interview. It is often recommended that each group ideally should be composed of individuals who are strangers to each other to avoid biases and to avoid the formation of sub-groups conducting conversations between themselves. However, as Morgan points out, the rigid application of this 'rule' would make it very difficult to conduct focus groups in a number of situations (Morgan and Krueger 1993), for example within organizations such as general practices, or within small communities. The most important design strategy to address this issue is to rely on a trained moderator to meet the potential problems posed by groups of acquaintances rather than to avoid them altogether (Morgan and Krueger 1993).

Snowball sampling involves asking respondents to pass details of the research and contact numbers on to other individuals who may be willing to participate. This method of sampling is particularly relevant when the individuals being studied may be known to each other, but not accessible through any known sampling list. Examples may include gay men and illegal drug users and groups whose confidentiality would be compromised if they were sampled through their medical records, e.g. immunization 'refusers' or users of complementary therapies.

The term 'theoretical sampling' which is often referred to in qualitative research does not, as may be supposed, distinguish it from 'actual sampling'. It is an approach whereby the purpose of the research (such as developing a theory or explanation) guides the sampling and data collection procedure. An initial set of observations or interviews will be conducted and analysed to guide the next stage of the research, which may include modifications in approach or sampling, in response to initial findings and the development of the explanation. One of the ways in which observational methods and semi-structured interviewing differ from quantitative methods is that it is entirely acceptable (indeed, it is seen as a strength of the method) to make adjustments to the sampling procedure while the data is being collected. This is possible because fieldwork and analysis take place concurrently and issues which arise from the analysis can be explored further and tested by, for example, recruiting more of a particular type of patient or observing specific clinics.

Data collection

A report of qualitative research should state how the interviewer or fieldworker presented themselves in the setting. In much health and health services research it is important that the researcher is known to be independent of the medical setting. This is particularly true if respondents are encouraged to speak openly about features of their health care. An assurance of confidentiality may be insufficient to avoid the problem since patients may be swayed by their interlocutor's (real or supposed) professional identity. If more than one interviewer or fieldworker was used, issues of comparability should be considered.

The importance of a well trained moderator in group interviewing has been stated already, but is worth emphasizing in the context of data collection. The transcription of group interview recordings is rendered virtually impossible if several people within the group talk simultaneously resulting in the loss of sections of data for analysis. A skilled facilitator should be able to minimize the occurrence of this as well as tactfully encouraging quiet members to contribute while restraining dominant ones (Krueger 1994).

Where recordings are made transcriptions can be made at several levels of detail. To transcribe the entire data set at a level suitable for conversational analysis (every utterance and pause precisely documented) will be inappropriately thorough for many research purposes. It may not be considered important to transcribe fully all of the interviewers statements, although her/his prompts and explanations will often be consequential in the analysis. The number of seconds taken up in a pause, or the length of a sigh or burst of laughter are all potentially important additions to the transcript and will often be considered necessary detail. As the analysis progresses it may be decided that certain sections of the interview do not need to be fully transcribed. Whenever feasible, all original recordings should be retained as unedited tapes, so that independent verification of the transcripts is possible.

Anonymized tape recordings and detailed fieldnotes may provide valuable material for subsequent analysis, perhaps in the light of new theoretical developments (Weaver 1994) or in combination with comparable data sets. There is considerable potential for secondary analysis of qualitative data, for which central archives are now available.

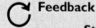

Feedback

Study design
It is important that qualitative methods be used for qualitative questions, such as 'How do patients perceive their care?' or 'Why are individuals unwilling to permit their children to be vaccinated?' The methods must be appropriate to the questions. For certain topics, group interviews may be better than individual sessions. Some information may only be revealed by one of the techniques of observation.

Sampling method
As you can see, the aim of sampling in qualitative research is different from that in quantitative research. Rather than seeking a sample that will represent the whole population, you attempt to obtain one that will provide either a broad range of views, or particular insights, or both.

Method of collecting data

Data collection is concerned with obtaining the true, unbiased views of subjects. Interviewers must be carefully trained to avoid prejudicing the responses obtained. It may be appropriate to include reference to the subjects' behaviour during interviews or focus groups (their facial expression or gestures, for instance). This can help with interpretation later.

Analysis

Having obtained your data, the next stage is analysis. The data must be examined, coded and tested to determine whether they are valid. This final activity will examine these processes and consider techniques that can help to ensure reliability and validity of the results.

 Activity 15.4

Read the extract below from Ziebland and Wright (1997). As you read, write short answers to the following questions.

1 What is the purpose of coding qualitative data?
2 What is textual analysis?
3 What methods can be used during the analysis of qualitative data to ensure reliability and validity?

 Analysing qualitative data

Coding is an essential part of qualitative data analysis, but is quite a different procedure from the coding stage of survey research. In qualitative analysis the coding is concerned with the relationship between chunks of data and categories or emerging themes, whereas in survey research it will involve the substitution of numerical codes for responses (e.g. 1 for 'yes'; 2 for 'no'; 3 for 'don't know'). The object of coding textual data from interview transcripts or fieldnotes is to ensure that all of the data which is relevant to each category can be identified and examined . . .

Traditional methods of qualitative data analysis have relied heavily on coloured pens, card systems, filing cabinets and cutting and pasting. The methods are undoubtedly laborious, but certainly retain contact with the data in its raw state, which could be a spur to creativity. The availability of word-processing packages (especially in Windows) has offered considerable advantages to researchers using textual data. Coding and retrieval of text is simplified through word-processing 'search' techniques and a split screen facilitates gathering, copying and pasting chunks of text into different files.

Word processors can be enormously helpful in searching large amounts of text for specific terms. The frequency with which particular words or phrases appear in a piece of text is of interest in some areas of research; for example, analysis of political speeches and mass media research. Content analysis of this sort requires an unambiguous, predefined coding system and aims to produce counts which may be tabulated and analysed using standard statistical techniques. It is distinct from the techniques of qualitative analysis in which data is coded or indexed in order to ensure that nothing relevant is lost to subsequent examination, not to reduce it to frequencies or cells in a table. This difference in analytic approach results from the theory building focus of interpretative research for which predefined coding, counting and tests of statistical significance are simply not germane.

Computer-assisted analysis

The evolution of computer software for analysing qualitative data has been welcomed as an important development with the potential to improve the rigour of analysis (Kelle 1995). The current software offers functions which enable more complex organization and retrieval of data than that possible with word-processing software.

Recent packages which have been designed to assist in the analysis of unstructured textual data all have 'code and retrieval' functions and several other uses which will be recognizable to researchers. These include the ability to define variables which can be used for selective retrievals (e.g. to examine separately by gender or age group excerpts referring to a particular phenomenon); to use algorithms to identify co-occurring codes in a range of logically overlapping or nesting possibilities; to attach comments and theoretical notes to sections of the text as 'memos'; to add new codes if and when required and join together existing codes. Most of the packages also provide counts of code frequencies.

These functions are all concerned with organizing and accessing the data, which are only the initial stages in qualitative analysis. It has also been suggested that computer-assisted analysis can help the researcher to build theoretical links, search for exceptions and examine 'crucial cases' where counter-evidence might be anticipated. A systematic search for 'disconfirming evidence' can be assisted by using Boolean operators (such as OR, AND, NOT) to examine the data. An examination of the context of the fragments may be achieved either through considering which other codes are attached to the data or by displaying the immediate context of the extract by including the lines of text which surround it. This function should particularly appeal to researchers who are concerned about the decontextualization which can result from fragmenting the data into coded chunks. The Hypersoft package (Dey 1993) uses what the developer calls 'hyperlinks' to capture the conceptual links which are observed between sections of the data, and protect the narrative structure from fragmentation.

There are many potential benefits to using a software package to help with the more laborious side of textual analysis but, as ever, some caution is advisable. One of the criticisms which is levelled at qualitative researchers is that the samples are too small and unrepresentative: the prospect of computer-assisted analysis may persuade researchers (or their funders) that they can manage much larger amounts of data and increase the 'power' of their study. Qualitative studies, which are not designed to be representative in terms of statistical generalizability, may gain little from an expanded sample size except a more cumbersome data set. The nature and size of the sample should be directed by the research question and analytic requirements, not by the available software. In some circumstances, a single case study design may be the most successful way of generating theory. Lee and Fielding (1995) warn against the assumption that using a computer package will make analysis less time-consuming, although it is hoped that it may make the process more demonstrably systematic. The essential tasks of studying the text, recognizing and refining the concepts, and coding the data are inescapably the work of the researcher. A computer package may be useful for gathering together chunks of data, establishing links between the fragments, organizing and reorganizing the display and helping to find exceptions, but no package is capable of perceiving a link or defining an appropriate structure for the analysis.

Testing the validity of the findings

In addition to the methods mentioned above (e.g. systematically searching for disconfirming evidence within the data) two other approaches are widely recommended to address the validity of the findings. These are 'triangulation' and 'respondent validation'. It is important to note that these will only be applicable in some circumstances. Silverman goes further and suggests these methods are 'usually inappropriate to qualitative research' (Silverman 1993: 156).

Triangulation

Ethnographic observation often includes a degree of triangulation in that multiple sources of data collection (e.g. direct participation, observation, informant and respondent interviews, etc.) are used. A study design which relies on interviews as the primary method may benefit from using other sources, such as a surveyor a review of case notes or a combination of group and individual interviews. However, as Hammersley and Atkinson have pointed out: 'one should not adopt a naively "optimistic" view that the aggregation of data from different sources will unproblematically add up to produce a more complete picture' (Hammersley and Atkinson 1983: 199). The problem is that different methods do sometimes produce different results and 'rarely does the inaccuracy of one approach to the data complement the accuracies of another' (Fielding and Fielding 1986: 35).

Respondent validation

Once the researcher has drawn tentative results from the data, they may choose to go back to the respondents and refine their findings in the light of their comments. In some research settings this will not be feasible. Fielding and Fielding recognize that the respondent may be able to clarify points and provide additional information about the context of their actions, but 'there is no reason to assume that members have privileged status as commentators on their actions. Such feedback cannot be taken as direct validation or refutation of the observer's inferences. Rather such processes of so-called "validation" should be treated as yet another source of data and insight' (Fielding and Fielding 1986: 43).

Respondent validation of group interviews may be achieved through conducting a small number of individual interviews with members of the focus groups, or running follow-up focus groups with the original participants to discuss the findings (Morgan 1993).

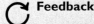 **Feedback**

1 When coding qualitative data, you should aim to identify all items of data that are present in your observations or in the records of your interviews. You should then attempt to determine which items are related to each other, in order to detect any emerging patterns between them. For example, if you wish to examine patients' satisfaction with the way that information is communicated to them, you may find them mentioning such themes as:

- lack of approachability of staff ('I didn't feel that I could ask him any questions')
- appearance of indifference ('She didn't seem to want to know what I thought')
- jargon ('I couldn't understand the words they used')

Ideally, you should try to ensure that no data are left out.

2 Textual analysis is a process of searching textual data for specific words or phrases. The aim is to identify the concepts present in the material and discover the relationships between them. The key words or phrases are detected (by eye or by computer) and coded. Their context may be deduced from the surrounding text.

3 The following techniques may help to ensure reliability and validity of qualitative findings:

- *search the data for 'disconfirming evidence'* – inconsistencies
- *use triangulation* – that is, different sources of data, or different methods to examine the same question; if the results are similar, this provides supporting evidence for their validity
- *Review your findings with some of the original subjects* – This is called respondent validation, and may enable you to obtain a deeper understanding of the concepts and their relationships

Summary

Qualitative methods are concerned with how people behave and how social systems operate in a natural context. They may be used to inquire about how or why people behave in particular ways. They can also investigate people's beliefs and their reasons for holding them. Qualitative methods are ideal for evaluating patient satisfaction when it is not possible to state in advance precisely which aspects are most important.

It is possible to use qualitative methods to help in planning a quantitative study, or to help interpret the results of a quantitative study. Qualitative methods may be based upon observation – on participant or non-participant observation, or upon interviewing – individual or group interviews, focus groups or nominal groups. Observation allows the researcher to discover what people do as well as what they say. Participant observation allows the researcher to become immersed in the surroundings of the subject and have a richer experience of the subject's life. It is important to realize that the practice of observing someone's behaviour may cause that behaviour to change (the Hawthorne effect). Interviewing allows a much deeper exploration of a topic. It is possible to ask standard questions and obtain information that may be more representative of the population. Some topics are very private and are more suited to individual interviews (e.g. sexuality). Some topics are sensitive and it may be better to undertake a semi-structured interview, allowing the interviewee to influence the discussion. Certain topics (such as dissatisfaction with nursing care) may be better approached using one of the group interview techniques.

Part of the process of analysis involves examining the data to determine whether they are valid. There are a number of techniques, such as the search for disconfirming evidence, triangulation and respondent validation.

References

Dey I (1993) *Qualitative data analysis: a user friendly guide for social scientists.* London: Routledge.

Dowell J, Huby G and Smith C (1996) *Scottish consensus statement on qualitative research in primary health care.* Dundee: Tayside Centre for General Practice.

Fielding N and Fielding J (1986) *Linking data,* qualitative research methods series no.4. London: Sage.

Fontana A and Frey JH (1994) Interviewing: the art of science, in Denzin NK and Lincoln YS (eds) *Handbook of qualitative research.* Thousand Oaks, CA: Sage.

Goffman E (1961) *Asylums.* Harmondsworth: Penguin.

Hammersley M, Atkinson P. (1983) Ethnography: principles in practice. London: Tavistock Publications.

Jones J and Hunter D (1995) Consensus methods for medical and health services research. *British Medical Journal* 311: 376–80.

Kelle U (ed.) (1995) *Computer aided qualitative data analysis theory, methods and practice.* London: Sage.

Kitzinger J (1995) Introducing focus groups. *British Medical Journal* 311: 299–302.

Krueger RA (1994) *Focus groups: A practical guide for applied research.* Thousand Oaks, CA: Sage.

Lee RL (1993) *Doing research on sensitive topics.* London: Sage.

Lee R and Fielding N (1995) User's experiences of qualitative data analysis software, in Kelle U (ed.) *Computer aided qualitative data analysis.* London: Sage.

Lofland J and Lofland LH (1984) *Analysing social settings,* 2nd edn. Belmont, CA: Wadsworth.

Merton RK and Kendall PL (1946) The focused interview. *American Journal of Sociology* 51: 541–57.

Moore CM (1994) Group techniques for team building. Thousand Oaks, CA: Sage.

Morgan DL (1988) *Focus groups as qualitative research.* London: Sage.

Morgan DL (ed.) (1993) Future directions for focus groups, in Morgan DL (ed.) *Successful focus groups: advancing the state of the art.* Newbury Park, CA: Sage.

Morgan DL and Krueger RA (1993) When to use focus groups and why, in Morgan DL (ed.) *Successful focus groups: advancing the state of the art.* Newbury Park, CA: Sage.

Pope C and Mays N (1995) Opening the black box: an encounter in the corridors of health services research. *British Medical Journal* 306: 315–18.

Rosenhan DL (1973) On being sane in insane places. *Science* CLXXIX: 250–8.

Roth J (1963) *Timetables: structuring the passage of time in hospital treatment and other careers.* Indianapolis, IN: Bobbs Merrill Co.

Silverman D (1993) *Interpreting qualitative data.* London: Sage.

Strong P (1979) *The ceremonial order of the clinic.* London: Routledge & Kegan Paul.

Weaver A (1994) Deconstructing dirt and disease: the case of TB, in Taraborrelli P (ed.) *Qualitative studies in health and medicine.* Aldershot: Avebury.

Ziebland S and Wright L (1997) Qualitative research methods, in Jenkinson C (ed.) *Assessment and evaluation of health and medical care.* Buckingham: Open University Press.

SECTION 6

Evaluating equity

Defining equity

Overview

Now you have examined the effectiveness, efficiency and humanity of health care interventions, it is still necessary to consider how to make effective health care available to all members of the community in an equitable way. Equity refers to the fair distribution of health services among groups or individuals. While it may be easy to define equity, is it more difficult to decide what is fair and just in practice, and how to implement these principles. Evaluative research plays an important role in this process as it informs decisions on how resources should be redistributed to improve equity. Equity depends on the concept of fairness. However, there are different ways of deciding how to distribute health care fairly. These may be described in terms of a number of ethical theories. This chapter will introduce some of the more common ethical theories relating to distributive justice, as well as the concepts of horizontal and vertical equity.

Learning objectives

By the end of this chapter you should be better able to:

- **explain the concept of fairness in the allocation of health care**
- **describe common theories of distributive justice (ethical theories)**
- **explain the concepts of horizontal and vertical equity**

Key terms

Equity Fairness, defined in terms of equality of opportunity, provision, use or outcome.

Horizontal equity The equal treatment of individuals or groups in the same circumstances.

Vertical equity The principle that individuals who are unequal should be treated differently according to their level of need.

What is equity?

Equity includes the concepts of fairness, justice and equality. It is assessed by comparing levels of health, or the ability of individuals and communities to obtain health care. There are two forms of equity. *Horizontal equity* refers to equal treatment for equal needs, the devotion of equal resources to patients with similar conditions, or equal access to care for people with equal needs. Donaldson and Gerard (1992) describe this as: i) providing equal *resources* for people with equal needs, allocating health service budgets to districts on the basis of population age, sex and standardized mortality ratio; ii) providing equal *access* to health care for people with equal need – for example, providing specialist units such as cancer units to treat those with similar illnesses, or adjusting waiting lists so that those with the same health care needs wait for the same length of time; iii) equal *utilization* of health care by those with equal need, such as ensuring similar length of hospital stay for similar conditions; iv) providing equal health aimed at reducing inequalities in health status between populations.

Vertical equity refers to unequal treatment for unequal needs, i.e. treating individuals who are unequal in society in different ways in order to overcome the effects of differences in their social or clinical situation. There are two ways of achieving vertical equity. In the first perspective (Mooney and Jan 1997) vertical equity requires that individuals with more need should have more treatment to bring them up to the same level as others with less need. This might include devoting more resources to patients with serious conditions than to those with trivial conditions or financing health care according to the ability to pay (Donaldson and Gerard 1992). An alternative perspective points out that equal use for equal need does not necessarily always result in unequal use for unequal need. If (as is described in the extract below) mildly hypertensive men are treated in the same way regardless of gender, age or ethnicity, but severely hypertensive men are more likely to receive treatment than severely hypertensive women, then equal use for equal need (horizontal equity) occurs for mild hypertension but not for severe hypertension (where there is vertical inequity). The following extract from Raine (2002) will describe these concepts in more detail.

Bias measuring bias

Once issues around the definition of need have been resolved, it must then be recognised that differences in health care use are not biased if they are due to differences in need. Such differences demonstrate unequal but fair care. The fair distribution of health care should be considered from two, related, perspectives. The first is that people with equal needs should be treated the same (equal use for equal need). This is referred to as the achievement of horizontal equity. For example, if we consider differences in clinical need, such as differences in disease severity or in co-morbidity, then patients with similar levels of disease severity should be equally likely to receive an effective intervention regardless of, for example, age or gender. The alternative perspective is that people with greater clinical needs should have more treatment than those with lesser needs (unequal use for unequal need) (Mooney and Jan 1997). This is referred to as the achievement of vertical equity. Thus, patients with severe disease should be more likely to receive an effective intervention compared with patients with a milder form of the same disease, regardless of age or gender. Although these perspectives of fairness are logically linked, it cannot be assumed that one follows the other as night follows day. Demonstration of equal use for equal need does not necessarily indicate unequal use for unequal need. This is because it cannot be *assumed* that equal use occurs at every level of need. For example, men and women with mildly elevated blood pressure may be equally likely to receive antihypertensive drugs (demonstrating equal use for equal need). But, although men with severe hypertension may be more likely to receive medication compared with men with mildly elevated blood pressure, the likelihood of medication for women may not vary according to degree of abnormality. Unequal use for unequal need occurs for men but not for women. This is unfair because the likelihood of treatment depends on disease severity, but it is not the same in men and women.

It is essential to take account of different levels of clinical need in order to measure the fair use of health care from both perspectives. Studies of bias vary in the extent to which they have examined fairness comprehensively. Some research has simply compared the utilisation of services by different groups, without any adjustment for differences in need between the groups (Chandra *et al.* 1998). Insofar as these studies are addressing the question of equal use for equal need, they are assuming that each individual, whatever their severity of ill-health, has an equal need for health care. More sophisticated studies adjust for need in order to examine the extent to which fairness is achieved (Raine 2000; Siassi and Messer 1976; Alexander and Sehgal 1998). The usual approach is to use multivariate analysis to examine whether need is the principal determinant of utilisation after controlling for other relevant factors (such as age, ethnic, economic group or gender). Let us return to our example where clinical need is measured in terms of disease severity, and the group of concern is men compared with women, to show how multivariate analysis, when used alone, can lead to misleading conclusions. When no gender difference in health service use is found after adjusting for need, this is said to reflect fair health care use. It is *assumed* that at every level of need (from mild to severe disease), the gender difference in health service use is the same. Specifically, equal use for equal need has been implicitly assumed. As I have shown, further analysis is required to test this assumption and to investigate whether the lack of a gender difference does occur for patients with both mild and severe disease.

Activity 16.1 will give you an opportunity to use the concepts of horizontal and vertical equity (based on the Mooney and Jan definition).

Activity 16.1

Which form of equity, horizontal or vertical, is addressed by the following?

1 Means-tested user fees.
2 Health status survey of 30–40-year-old dialysis patients from five renal centres.
3 Progressive taxation.
4 Clinical guidelines for maximum length of stay in hospital after uncomplicated herniotomy.
5 Planning spatial distribution of primary health care centres.
6 Resource allocation to regions using standardized mortality ratios.
7 Nutrition support for children in deprivation areas.
8 Comparing waiting lists for hip replacement between districts.

Feedback

Numbers 1, 3 and 7 address Mooney and Jan's definition of vertical equity, while 2, 4, 5, 6 and 8 address horizontal equity. However, remember that Raine's definition of vertical equity requires consideration of equal use within each level of need for the social group under consideration.

While most people would agree with the definitions cited above, it is less easy to decide what is fair or just in practice. The next section looks at principles that have been developed to aid such decisions and inform their implementation.

Ethical theories

Defining equity is relatively easy. The difficulty comes in deciding what is fair or just. Most of the health and health care issues related to equity come under the category of 'distributive justice' – that is, how benefits, resources and burdens of society are distributed to each individual. The rules of each theory define how society cooperates and these relate directly to the values that a society holds. Theories of distributive justice differ in the type of rules that they purport. Some examples might include:

- to each person an equal share;
- to each person according to individual needs;
- to each person according to individual efforts;
- to each person according to societal contributions;
- to each person according to merit.

Theories of distributive justice can be broadly divided into libertarian, liberal and collectivist. The next few sections will briefly consider each of these in relation to health care.

Libertarian theory

Libertarians believe in the protection of individual freedom (e.g. political liberty, free speech and economic freedom). The contemporary theoretical foundation for libertarian theory is based on the work of Nozick. He advocates the minimal state and the free market, which protects individual liberty. Nozick's theory states that people are entitled to what they have, provided it was acquired justly. For example, he argues that for the state to tax individual people in order to provide goods and services for the least advantaged class is a form of theft by the state against the private individual. In Britain, the NHS changes of the early 1990s introduced a market-based health system, which grew out of the belief in the pre-eminence of individual liberty. Other countries around the world followed a similar principle. However, one obvious limitation to libertarian theory is that biological and genetic influences mean that the distribution of *health* cannot be described as fair. This has implications for the allocation of *health care* under a libertarian system.

Liberal theory

Liberal theory also emphasizes individual liberty, but also includes the concept of 'need' in its definition. Like libertarian theory, liberal theory relies on the free market to allocate resources, but also recognizes the unequal distribution of assets. State intervention is therefore deemed appropriate when the market fails to safeguard the needs of all the members of society. One type of liberal theory, known as utilitarianism, argues that there is a moral obligation to achieve the greatest good for the greatest number and places primary importance on efficiency. Utilitarianism has sometimes been called unjust because it could justify harm if this maximizes total utility. Public health interventions such as universal immunization for measles or polio are based on utilitarian principles.

An alternative type of liberal theory argues that we should maximize the income and wealth of the least well off sectors of society. Goods should therefore be equally distributed unless unequal distribution is to the advantage of the least favoured groups. This is sometimes called the 'maximin' principle (a term adopted by Rawls). This theory is based on the assumption that if people did not know their position in society they would opt to maximize the position of the worst off. This type of theory supports the idea of the welfare state. However, it can be difficult to implement as in practice societies do not always adhere to the maximin principle.

Collectivist theory

Collectivist theories are based on three main goals: equality, freedom and fraternity, though the dominant concern is equality. Collectivist theories are therefore egalitarian and favour positive, equalizing measures to redistribute rights and wealth. Socialists, for example, would argue that the market system can be used to achieve these egalitarian aims whereas Marxists would argue that the system is inherently in conflict with these goals and it is therefore necessary to give the state the primary role in production and allocation.

The NHS in the UK was originally founded on egalitarian principles. It was set up in 1948 and was intended to achieve equity in using and distributing resources. This included equity of initial access to the health care system and equity in terms of quality and quantity of services once access had been achieved.

 Activity 16.2

Application of each of these approaches would have different consequences for health care provision. Consider a vaccination programme against a disease such as polio for a population where the vaccination is believed to be effective for all children. How would libertarian, liberal and collectivist approaches differ in their approach to vaccination?

 Feedback

There is no single answer to how each philosophical standpoint would address the issue of vaccination, but we can hypothesize about some possible alternatives.

Libertarian theory places emphasis on the individual. A health system that is based on libertarian values may not be publicly funded. People with the means to pay for health care are able to pay for vaccination. However, those without adequate means may not be able to pay for vaccination.

Liberal theory recognizes the unequal distribution of assets and so state intervention is deemed appropriate when the market fails to address the needs of all members of society. A liberal approach such as utilitarian theory would advocate universal immunization of every child in the population. The vaccination policy of the NHS is based on this type of approach.

Collectivist theory emphasizes egalitarian goals. Collectivists might argue that the utilitarian is making judgements about the welfare of children based on his or her own value judgements. Factors other than the avoidance of disease may be important to some individuals, such as the risk of adverse effects from the vaccine. Arguably the ability to benefit should be judged by the patient (or in this example, his or her parent) depending on their personal values regarding health.

Summary

This chapter has allowed you to consider alternative views of what constitutes fairness in allocation of health care. Equity describes the concepts of fairness, justice and equality. Horizontal equity involves equal treatment of those with equal need (however defined). Vertical equity seeks to provide greater resources to those who are disadvantaged in society, though it is also necessary to then ensure equal use for each social group at each level of need. A number of ethical theories exist to help determine which acts are right or wrong and which are fair or unfair. Different societies and individuals base their decision-making on different ethical theories. Many people act in accordance with the principles of one of these ethical theories without being aware of doing so.

The following types of theory may be applied within the context of health care. A health care system based on libertarian theory emphasizes the role of the free market in protecting individual freedom and ensuring efficiency. It would not take account of the fact that health need is not distributed equally. A health care system base on a liberal theory such as utilitarianism essentially seeks to produce the greatest health gain for a given amount of resources. It would not necessarily seek to distribute this health gain to those in greatest need in the community. A health care system based on collectivist theory would emphasize egalitarian principles and emphasizes equality and freedom. This is the type of principle on which the NHS was founded.

References

Alexander G and Sehgal A (1998) Barriers to cadaveric renal transplantation among Blacks, women and the poor. *Journal of the American Medical Association* 280: 1148–52.

Chandra NC, Ziegelstein RC, Rogers WJ, Tiefenbrunn AJ, Gore JM, French WJ *et al.* (1998) Observations of the treatment of women in the United States with myocardial infarction. *Archives of Internal Medicine* 158: 981–8.

Donaldson C and Gerard K (1992) *Economics of health care financing: the visible hand.* London: Macmillan.

Mooney G and Jan S. (1997) Vertical equity: weighting outcomes or establishing procedures? *Health Policy* 39: 79–87.

Raine R (2000) Is there really gender bias in health care use? *Journal of Health Services Research and Policy* 5: 237–49.

Raine R. (2002) Bias measuring bias. *Journal of Health Services Research and Policy* 7: 65–7.
Siassi I and Messer S (1976) Psychotherapy with patients from lower socioeconomic groups. *American Journal of Psychotherapy* 30: 29–40.

17 Assessing equity

Overview

In the previous chapter, you examined some ethical theories that justify different concepts of 'what is fair'. In this chapter you will see how equity can be operationalized for the purpose of health care evaluation. First you will consider the relationship between equity and need, what definitions to use and what variables to measure. Specific examples are given of the problems of measuring equity by access and by utilization. Finally, the chapter guides you through the different steps of evaluating equity.

Learning objectives

By the end of this chapter you should be better able to:

- **explain the relationship between the concepts of equity and need**
- **outline the study designs and analytical methods that can be used to evaluate equity**

Key terms

Normative need A professional assessment of a person's need for health care based on objective measures.

How to measure equity

Assessing whether a service is equitable involves measuring and comparing several dimensions. These include: inputs (such as staff per population, hospital beds per population, expenditure); process (use, such as hospital admission rates, consultation rates); and outcomes (mortality, health status, patient satisfaction). These measures can be compared between groups, but to assess whether the differences are *inequitable*, you have to relate the difference to clinical *need*.

How to integrate equity and need

The disciplines of sociology, psychology, philosophy and economics have all constructed a definition of 'need'. In the context of health care evaluation, normative need can be defined as 'the capacity to benefit from health care' (Stevens and

Gabbay 1991). It is only possible to benefit from health care that is effective. It stands to reason that those in poorest health have the greatest capacity to benefit from health care, provided that effective interventions exist.

The need for health care varies for many reasons, including the following:

1 *Geographical factors* – there are differences in the incidence and prevalence of many diseases between different countries or regions. For example, in the UK there are national variations in the rates of chronic liver disease (Prince *et al.* 2001).

2 *Socioeconomic factors* – the association between deprivation and poor health status has long been recognized. However, association between deprivation and health status occurs at all levels of the spectrum, not just among the most deprived (or the very affluent). For example, in the UK, the Whitehall Study (Marmot *et al.* 1984; Marmot and Shipley 1996) demonstrated differing rates of illness among different grades of civil servants. None of the civil servants could be described as deprived, yet there was still a health gradient such that the higher grade civil servants had better life expectancies than those of lower grades. This gradient persisted even after retirement.

3 *Ethnic factors* – the association between ethnicity and health is well established. For example, Caucasians are more likely to have cystic fibrosis while Africans may be more likely to have sickle cell disease.

4 *Age* – communities with a greater proportion of elderly people have a higher incidence of some diseases, for example cardiovascular disease (Maggioni *et al.* 1993).

5 *Sex* – some diseases are more likely to occur in men. For example, coronary heart disease (CHD) is more likely to cause death in men than in women (Rayner *et al.* 1998), though death rates from CHD in women are also high.

6 *Co-morbidities* – people with several coexisting diseases are likely to have a high need for health care. For example, a recent study found that in older patients with depression, patients had on average three other co-morbid conditions.

There are a number of variables that can be used to assess the need that a community has for health care. Assessing the age/sex structure of the population, and including the standardized mortality ratio (SMR), can give a useful if somewhat limited means of comparing the relative needs for health services of different communities. Standardized instruments can also be used to assess need. For example, measures such as the Charlson Index (Charlson *et al.* 1987) or the Index of Coexistent Disease (Greenfield *et al.* 1993) (see Chapter 3) could be used to assess co-morbidity. Measures of severity could also be used to assess need, for example the New York Heart Association Classification (Criteria Committee of the New York Heart Association 1964) is widely used to assess need in cardiac patients (although its psychometric attributes have not been fully assessed). There are several indices that can be used to assess socioeconomic status. In the UK, occupation is sometimes used as a proxy for socioeconomic status (e.g. the system developed by the Office for National Statistics 2000). Other systems use place of residence to indicate social class (Jarman 1984). However, these systems may not be entirely appropriate for use with some populations, such as elderly people. They are also unlikely to translate to developing country contexts.

Which study design is appropriate?

A randomized design is not usually used to examine equity because the variables of interest, like age and sex, are the very factors which randomization is designed to ensure are distributed equally among the intervention and control groups. So, for example, it would not make sense to investigate equity of access to a health care intervention among old versus young people using a randomized design where people are randomly assigned to receive the intervention. Instead, an observational study design to examine the extent to which equity occurs in practice is usually used, for example, a cohort or an ecological study (see Chapters 8 and 9). An exception would be the measurement of equity of health outcomes, which could be examined in a randomized design (e.g. the extent to which a randomly assigned intervention produces health improvement in men versus women).

Within these designs, there are several ways in which adjustment is made for levels of need. The simplest method is to use a ratio of use to need, or of access to need. However, this method does not take account of potential confounding factors. A more commonly used approach is multivariable analysis. This is a useful method which allows measurement of use having adjusted for clinical need and for potential confounding factors.

There are two ways of investigating the modifying effect of indicators of clinical need on health care use in the groups of concern (e.g. the old versus the young). These are either to examine interactions between the social factor of concern (e.g. age), and a measure of clinical need, or to stratify analyses according to different levels of need. These analyses would indicate whether vertical inequity was present.

However, before you can collect the data, you need to operationalize these concepts. The following reading illustrates several ways of defining equity and will guide you in selecting the appropriate definitions for health care evaluation.

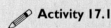 **Activity 17.1**

Read the following extract from Mooney (1983) that outlines seven possible ways of defining equity. This passage contains the Latin expression *ceteris paribus*. It means 'if all other things are equal'. Consider the seven definitions of equity in health care. What do you understand each of them to mean?

1   Equality of expenditure per capita.
2   Equality of inputs (resources) per capita.
3   Equality of input for equal need.
4   Equality of access for equal need.
5   Equality of utilization for equal need.
6   Equality of marginal met need.
7   Equality of health.

📖 Seven definitions of equity

1 Equality of expenditure per capita

This definition would suggest that if the budget available for health care were allocated to different regions, say, pro rata with the size of the regional population then this would result in an equitable allocation. Indeed whatever the definition of equity the relative size of the groups for which equity is being pursued is likely to be a major determinant of an equitable distribution.

2 Equality of inputs (resources) per capita

If the prices of different resources (e.g. land) vary across different regions then a second view of equity would suggest that those regions with higher than average prices should not be penalised as would be the case with the first definition. In other words, allowance should be made for differential prices so that the resources (labour, land and capital) which can be purchased with the allocated expenditure are the same per capita. Thus relatively high priced regions would receive more (and vice versa for low priced areas) under this definition than under the first.

3 Equality of input for equal need

Variations in need, beyond simple population size, are explicitly recognised in this definition. For example, it can be argued that the age/sex structure influences the health needs of the population (children and the elderly tend to need more hospital beds than do the middle-aged; the need for gynaecological beds is clearly related to the size of the female population); the greater the morbidity in a population the greater the health care resources it merits; marital status of the population – the divorced, separated and widowed have a higher utilisation rate of psychiatric beds than the married; the extent of patient flows into and out of various regions; and so on. Thus if it were possible to say that for one population its 'need' was 10% greater than that of another of the same size then under this definition, *ceteris paribus*, that population would receive 10% more resources than the other.

4 Equality of (opportunity of) access for equal need

If as in section 3 above, inputs are allocated pro rata with beds, it might be argued that this was not equitable in those areas faced with high costs (as opposed to prices) of delivering health care. For example, to provide the same level of service can be more expensive in rural areas than in urban areas. Domiciliary services such as health visiting and district nursing are likely to involve more travelling time in rural than in urban areas. Patients in rural areas normally have higher costs to bear *either* in travel, inconvenience, etc. *or* in forgoing health benefits by not being treated at all or accepting potentially lower quality care locally. Hospitals serving remote areas are likely to have to bear higher costs (e.g. maternity cases from remote areas are admitted well before the due date). In effect, defining equity in this way is adjusting the definition under section 3 to make allowance for these differential costs. Equal access is thus defined as equal costs *to patients*, although it should be noted that where there is not equality of access there may be effects on health service costs. These can be in the case of 'distant' or 'remote' patients, for example, both upward because of longer lengths of hospital stay and higher costs of community care or downward because of lower utilisation rates.

5 Equality of utilisation for equal need

Under section 4 above, if everyone's information, tastes and preferences for health and health care were the same, then equality of access for equal need should be the same as equality of utilisation for equal need. But individuals do differ with respect to these charac-teristics. People experience different thresholds of pain; some are more informed about health and health care matters; some are more ready to sit in GPs' surgeries than others or to travel long distances to receive care. Consequently it may be erroneous to assume that equality of access for equal need can be equated with equality of utilisation for equal need. Under a definition of equity based on equality of utilisation for equal need there may thus be a desire to discriminate positively in favour of those who are less willing to utilise health care.

Under this utilisation definition of equity it is important to consider the relationship between demand, supply and utilisation. Utilisation is a function of *both* supply and demand. If the supply side has been organised in such a way that there is equality of access for equal need (as in sec. 4) but not equality of utilisation for equal need, this means that the only remaining variable creating the inequity is demand. Behind the concept of demand lies that of satisfaction for the consumer/patient. The greater the utility an individual expects to obtain from a good the greater the amount he is willing to pay for it. What this means in terms of health care is that if we choose this fifth definition of equity in preference to the fourth we are arguing that individuals' demand for health care should be the same for equal need – given that they all face the same supply.

It is important to be aware of the type of judgments underlying this fifth definition. For example in the context of the multiply-deprived it might be suggested that it is not enough to attempt to provide equality of access for equal need. Given that even then they may not have as high a take-up rate as the non-multiply-deprived, additional resources should be made available to them i.e. in order to achieve equality of utilisation for equal need, there should be additional resources made available to multiply-deprived areas, more than in proportion to any extra need that exists.

6 Equality of marginal met need

Assuming (i) that regions rank needs in order of priority to be met (in the sense that, however defined, as they receive more and more resources, the additional needs they meet will be of lower and lower priority), and (ii) that the order of this ranking is the same across all regions, then, under this definition, equity would be achieved when each region with its available budget was just able to meet the same 'last' (or 'marginal') need. Put another way, equity would be achieved if each region would stop treating the same specific need if each of their budgets were cut by, say, £10 000.

7 Equality of health

All the earlier definitions have argued that if health needs varied then resources should as well. But providing resources in this type of way is in a sense a shoring-up operation i.e. resources are made available to try to cope to an equal extent with the problems arising. Unless all these problems are then cured there is no reason to believe that allocating resources pro rata with need will lead to equality of health across different regions.

If we argue that the goal of an equitable health service is to make the level of health the same in all regions and/or in all social classes, this requires *much* greater positive discrimin-ation than required by any of the input orientated definitions. Thus while all the earlier definitions tended to be concerned with equity in terms of the allocation of health care resources, the emphasis on health under this seventh definition would lead to a very unequal distribution of health service resources.

Feedback

1 Equality of expenditure per capita involves allocating the same health resources to every individual. For example, a health care budget might be allocated equally per person in the population. It makes no distinction between individuals in terms of their need for health care.

2 Equality of inputs per capita means allocating equal services to each individual, thus avoiding inequity arising because the cost of care (such as salaries) varies between places. There is still no distinction between individuals in terms of their need for health care.

3 Equality of input for equal need uses indicators of health needs (such as the age/sex structure of the population) to determine those sections of the population with greater requirements for health care. Extra resources are supplied to those sections of the population with greater measured need of health care. The main difficulty here is to obtain a formula that can quantify the differences in need. For example, since the 1970s the NHS has used formulae to promote a more equitable allocation of resources for hospital and community care. The Resource Allocation Working Party (RAWP) and its successors have recommended that money should be distributed on the basis of the size and age-sex distribution of an area's population, taking into account relative health needs as indicated by the standardized mortality ratio.

4 Equality of access (or supply) for equal need involves making equal services available to patients in equal need. More resources would be provided to improve the access of those sections of the population who incur the greatest personal cost in obtaining care, such as those living far from urban centres. Indicators of access could include availability of health care professionals, waiting times, or user charges.

5 Equality of utilization for equal need allows for the actual patterns of uptake of health care that occur in different communities. Utilization is influenced by the preferences, perceptions and prejudices of both patient and health care provider. For example, those communities which are more deprived may make less use of the health care that is available compared to more affluent communities.

6 Equality of marginal met need accepts that there are differences in the costs of meeting the same needs in different communities. This is best illustrated by the hypothetical example where all communities rank their health care needs in order, and all have the same list of needs. It would only be possible to achieve an equitable distribution of health resources by allocating resources to each community in whatever amounts are necessary for them all to provide the same items of care on their lists.

7 Equality of health assumes that it is not sufficient to provide greater amounts of health care to the more deprived communities, but that they should receive a disproportionately greater amount of resources in order to achieve the same health status as more affluent communities. Inequalities in health could arise from the level of resources, housing conditions, exposure to environmental hazards and different lifestyles and behaviours. Some influences on health are therefore avoidable (such as those due to lifestyle choices), but others are unavoidable (such as environmental exposure). The outcome of policies to address equality of health could be measured using a generic health instrument such as the SF-36.

It is usual to assess equity in terms of either access to, or utilization of, health care. In the literature these two terms are not often well defined and are sometimes confused. Activity 17.2 will help to explain the difference between equality of access and equality of utilization.

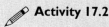 **Activity 17.2**

Read the following extract from Mooney (1983) and then try and describe the difference between equality of access and equality of utilization.

Access versus utilisation

The major distinction to be drawn between access and utilisation is that access is *wholly* a question of supply; utilisation is a function of both supply and demand (or need). Thus equal access for equal need occurs when individuals with the same needs face the same supply curve, i.e., the same costs *to themselves*. Thus two individuals living the same distance from a general practitioner's surgery and facing the same costs of attendance (e.g. both take their cars) have equal access to the general practitioner.

Less straightforwardly, equality of access can be achieved by taking some services to patients rather than vice versa. Thus specialists from major hospitals may not only run outpatient clinics in their own hospitals (normally based in densely populated areas) but also go out to smaller rural hospitals to hold outpatient clinics there. In this way the differential access problems created by distance can be reduced and perhaps even eliminated.

It is important to stress that equality of access is about equal *opportunity*: the question of whether or not the opportunity is exercised is not relevant to equity defined in terms of access. This cannot be said too strongly: it is lack of appreciation of this point which is at the root of much of the confusion that exists in comparing access and utilisation in equity in health care.

What of equality of utilisation? As indicated above utilisation is a function of supply *and* demand. Thus an individual's utilisation of health care facilities will depend not only on access (i.e. supply) but also on his or her perception of the benefits of care. Since individuals will differ in their perception of benefits . . . even if they have equal *access* to health care it does not follow that they will have equal utilisation. Furthermore, if equal utilisation is the goal, in some circumstances this will best be achieved by discriminating in terms of access.

Feedback

Mooney describes access in terms of 'supply'. He suggests that access to services can be made more equal by taking those services (such as a specialist clinic) into more distant or deprived areas. Equality of access is therefore about equality of opportunity to receive health care. It has nothing to do with whether individuals or communities actually take advantage of such opportunities. It is important to realize that access is not simply a matter of having the service in a convenient location. The community must know that it is available and that they might benefit from it.

Utilization is described in terms of both 'supply' and 'demand'. If the health care is made accessible to the community, people may still choose not to use it. Equality of utilization requires that those with the greatest need for care perceive that they have this need. It also requires that the health care on offer should provide them with the greatest benefits. In addition, they must have adequate access (see below) to enable them to take advantage of the care on offer.

Main steps in assessing equity

This section will describe the main steps that you will need to take in order to evaluate equity.

1 First, choose the definition of equity that you want to use. This will determine exactly what you will need to measure. For example, you may decide that you want to use a definition that addresses equal utilization for equal need. You would then need to measure utilization. Routine data may be helpful in assessing utilization and are often collected on a variety of procedures, such as surgical interventions, prescriptions and immunizations. Sometimes routine data include enough details of the patients to determine their social class and other indicators of general health needs such as age and sex. If routine data are not available, you could perform a survey specifically to collect these data, although this is likely to be quite expensive. Conducting a specific survey has the advantages of relating directly to the population that you wish to study, and collecting exactly those items of data that you require, using standardized definitions. These data are also more likely to be more accurate and complete.

2 Next, consider the population who will be served by the intervention that you are evaluating and the social group of concern in your study. This may be old people, or people from minority ethnic groups, for example.

3 To assess equity in terms of need, you should next estimate the specific need for the intervention. If the intervention is a drug treatment for a particular disease, you will need to identify the population who would benefit from the treatment (e.g. people with AIDS). This may be difficult. For example, for HIV national registration data is poor. This makes it difficult to identify all the people in the defined population who have the disease and who therefore need the drug treatment.

4 Now relate use to need. Here are some examples.

a) for coronary heart disease health promotion:

- assess need by using surveys of the prevalence of risk factors (e.g. smoking or obesity by social class)
- assess use by number of patients (e.g. white versus non-white patients) receiving health promotion information in health centres

b) for treatment in secondary care:

- assess need by using mortality statistics (e.g. from death certificates)
- assess use (e.g. among men versus women from hospital statistics)

c) for rehabilitation:

- assess need from hospital discharge data for specific diagnoses
- assess use of physiotherapy or occupational therapy among, for example, older and younger patients.

Simple analysis of this data would involve calculation of the ratio between need and use/access. However, it is more informative to use multivariable analysis as described earlier to evaluate equity having adjusted for need and potential confounding factors.

Summary

In this chapter you have seen how to operationalize equity for the purpose of health care evaluation. In practical terms, it is useful to distinguish between the following definitions:

- equality of expenditure per capita;
- equality of inputs (resources) per capita;
- equality of input for equal need;
- equality of access for equal need;
- equality of utilization for equal need;
- equality of marginal met need;
- equality of health.

You also looked in some detail at measures of access and use, and how these can be related to need. Finally, the chapter outlined the steps in designing a study to evaluate equity.

References

Charlson ME, Pompei P, Ales KL and McKenzie CR (1987) A new method of classifying prognostic comorbidity in longitudinal studies: development and validation. *Journal of Chronic Diseases* 40: 373–83.

Criteria Committee of the New York Heart Association (1964) *Diseases of the Heart and Blood Vessels: Nomenclature and Criteria for Diagnosis*, 6th edn. Boston, MA: Little, Brown.

Greenfield S, Apolone G, McNeil BJ and Cleary PD (1993) The importance of co-existent disease in the occurrence of postoperative complications and one-year recovery in patients undergoing total hip replacement: comorbidity and outcomes after hip replacement. *Medical Care* 31: 141–54.

Jarman B (1984) Underprivileged areas: validation and distribution of scores. *British Medical Journal* 289: 1587–92.

Maggioni AP, Maseri A, Fresco C, Franzosi MG, Mauri F, Santoro E and Tognoni G (1993) Age-related increase in mortality among patients with first myocardial infarctions treated with thrombolysis. The Investigators of the Gruppo Italiano per lo Studio della Sopravvivenza nell'Infarto Miocardico (GISSI-2). *New England Journal of Medicine* 329(20): 1442–8.

Marmot MG and Shipley MJ (1996) Do socioeconomic differences in mortality persist after retirement? 25 year follow up of civil servants from the first Whitehall study. *British Medical Journal* 313: 1177–80.

Marmot MG, Shipley MJ and Rose G (1984) Inequalities in death – specific explanations of a general pattern? *The Lancet* i: 1003–6.

Mooney G (1983) Equity in health care: confronting the confusion. *Effective Health Care* 1: 179–84.

Office for National Statistics (2000) *Standard Occupational Classification* 2000. London: The Stationery Office.

Prince MI, Chetwynd A, Diggle P, Jarner M, Metcalf JV and James OF (2001) The geographical distribution of primary biliary cirrhosis in well-defined cohort. *Hepatology* 34(6): 1083–8.

Rayner M, Mockford C and Boaz A (1998) *Coronary Heart Disease Statistics* (British Heart Foundation Statistics Database). London: British Heart Foundation.

Stevens A and Gabbay J (1991) Needs assessment needs assessment. *Health Trends* 23: 20–3.

Glossary

Autonomy The principle that human beings have free will and the right to make choices about their actions and about what happens to them.

Beneficence The principle of striving to do good.

Bias An error that results in a systematic deviation from the estimation of the association between exposure and outcome.

Capital cost The value of capital resources which have useful lives greater than one year.

Case-mix The mix of cases (or patients) that a provider cares for.

Causality The relating of causes to the effects they produce.

Confounding Situation in which an estimate of the association between a risk factor (exposure) and outcome is distorted because of the association of the exposure with another risk factor (a confounding variable) for the outcome under study.

Construct The hypothetical concept that a questionnaire or other type of instrument is intended to measure.

Controls A group of patients that do not receive the treatment that is under investigation.

Cost The value of resources usually expressed in monetary terms.

Cost-benefit analysis An economic evaluation technique in which outcomes are expressed in monetary terms.

Cost-effectiveness analysis Economic evaluations with outcomes measured in health units.

Cost minimization A method of economic analysis for comparing the costs of different interventions which produce the same outcome.

Cost-utility analysis Economic evaluations where the outcomes are measured in health units which capture not just the quantitative but also the qualitative aspects of the outome, such as quality of life.

Cross-sectional study A study design where exposure and outcome are measured at the same time.

Dignity The principle that human beings are worthy of respect and have the right to be treated with courtesy and with consideration for their feelings.

Direct costs Resources used in the design, implementation, receipt and continuation of a health care intervention.

Discount rate The rate at which future costs and outcomes are discounted to account for time preference.

Discounting A method for adjusting the value of costs and outcomes which occur in different time periods into a common time period, usually the present.

Disease-specific measures Instruments that focus on the particular aspects of the disease being studied.

Double blind When neither patients nor clinicians know the treatment to which patients have been allocated.

Ecological fallacy The effects measured in groups may not be applicable at the level of individuals.

Economic analysis A general term for a number of related techniques which seek to identify, measure, value and compare the costs and consequences of alternative actions.

Effectiveness The extent to which an intervention produces a beneficial result under usual conditions of clinical care.

Efficiency (cost-effectiveness) The cost of providing a health care intervention in relation to the improvement of health outcomes.

Equity Fairness, defined in terms of equality of opportunity, provision, use or outcome.

Ethnography A research method used in sociology and anthropology that systematically describes the culture of a group of people.

Evaluation The critical assessment of the value of an activity.

External validity (generalizability) The extent to which the results of a study can be generalized to the population from which the sample was drawn.

Financial (budgetary) costs The accounting cost of a good or service usually representing the original (historical) amount paid as distinct from the opportunity cost.

Fixed costs A cost of production that does not vary with the level of content.

Focus group A group interview including between 6 and 12 participants and a facilitator who guides the discussion to cover the research topics.

Generic measures Instruments that measure general aspects of a person's health, such as mobility, sleeping and appetite.

Hawthorne effect The tendency for the act of observing behaviour to change the behaviour that is being observed.

Health care Any activity that is intended to improve the state of physical, mental or social function of people.

Health-related quality of life The impact of the condition on the social functioning of a person, partly determined by the person's environment.

Horizontal equity The equal treatment of individuals or groups in the same circumstances.

Humanity The quality of being civil, courteous or obliging to others.

Impairment The physical signs of the condition (pathology), usually measured by clinicians.

Index measures Measures of health that include a number of different health dimensions and aggregates them into a single score.

Indirect costs The value of resources expended by patients and their carers to enable individuals to receive an intervention.

Intangible costs The costs of discomfort, pain, anxiety or inconvenience.

Intention to treat analysis When patients' results are analysed on the basis of the study arm to which they were randomly allocated irrespective of the treatment that they actually received.

Internal validity The extent to which the results of a study are not affected by bias and confounding.

Latency period The time interval between disease occurrence and detection.

Matching A technique used to adjust for the effects of confounding. Controls are selected in such a way that the distribution of potential confounders among the controls is similar to the cases.

Multiple groups Measurements of exposure and outcome are made on a number of groups at a single point in time.

Multiple time series A number of different groups are defined and measurements made at a number of points in time.

Nominal group technique A method of developing group consensus recorded in which participants first record their individual views on the topic, views are then discussed and then recorded privately again by each participant.

Non-maleficence The principle of avoiding harm.

Non-randomized (observational) study A study that examines the effects of health care without influencing the care that is provided or the patients who receive it.

Normative need A professional assessment of a person's need for health care based on objective measures.

Odds ratio The ratio of the odds of exposure in cases to the odds of exposure in controls.

Opportunity (economic) cost The value of the next best alternative forgone as a result of the decision made.

Participant observation Method of data collection in which the researcher participates in the process that is being studied, as well as acting as observer.

Placebo An inert medicine or procedure that can be given to the control group in an intervention study.

Profile measures Measures of health that include a number of health dimensions and produces a range of scores representing these different dimensions.

Prospective The patients and interventions (exposures) are identified in the present and followed up in the future to determine the outcomes.

Quality-adjusted life years (QALYs) A numerical representation of the value attached to a combination of quantity and quality of life, where one year of perfect health is set at "1".

Random sample A group of subjects selected from a population in a random manner (ie each member of the population has an equal chance of being selected).

Randomization The process of allocating patients to treatment based on chance. It is not possible for the investigator, clinician or patient to predict the allocation in advance.

Recurrent cost The value of recurrent resources with useful lives of less than one year that have to be purchased at least once a year.

Reliability The extent to which an instrument produces consistent results.

Responsiveness The extent to which an instrument detects real changes in the state of health of a person.

Restriction A technique to reduce the effects of a confounding variable by requiring that all study subjects either have this confounder or do not.

Retrospective The patients have already experienced the interventions (exposures) in the past and are followed up through to the present day.

Risk The proportion of individuals experiencing a particular outcome over a specified period of time.

Risk ratio The ratio of the risk of a given outcome from the treatment under investigation to the risk of the same outcome from the control treatment.

Sampling frame A list of the members of the population who would be eligible for inclusion in a study.

Single blind When patients do not know the treatment to which they have been allocated but clinicians do.

Single time-series One group (or population) is defined and measurements are made at a number of points in time.

Statistical association The demonstration that the outcome varies with the intervention that is being evaluated.

Statistical significance The likelihood that an association can be explained by chance alone.

Therapeutic equipoise Where the investigator, clinician and patient do not know which of the available interventions is most likely to be beneficial for the patient.

Time preference People's preference for consumption (or use of resources) now rather than later because they value present consumption more than the same consumption in the future.

Utility values Numerical representation of the degree of satisfaction with health status, health outcome or health care.

Validity The extent to which an instrument measures what it intends to measure.

Variable cost A cost of production that varies directly with the level of output.

Vertical equity Unequal treatment for unequal need; for example, investing greater resources in areas with greater need.

Index